W9-BGV-339

Dr. Scott JENSEN

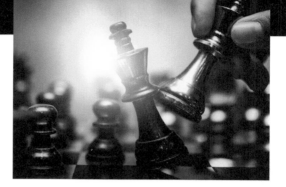

We've Been PLAYED...

Exposing the TRIAD of TYRANNY

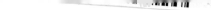

This book is dedicated to my grandchildren and their future freedom.

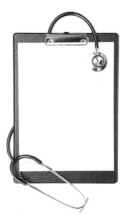

We've Been Played . . . Exposing the Triad of Tyranny

Copyright © 2022 by Scott Jensen

Published by Bronzebow Publishing
Minneapolis, Minnesota 55406

ISBN 978-0-9724563-4-0

All rights reserved. No part of this publication may be reproduced, stored in a retrieval system, or transmitted in any means—electronic, mechanical, digital, photocopy, recording, or any other—except for brief quotations in printed reviews, without the prior permission of the publishers.

First printing May 2022
10 9 8 7 6 5 4 3 2 1

Printed in the United States of America

table of
contents

"The truth is **INCONTROVERTIBLE.** Malice may attack it, ignorance may deride it, but in the end, there it is."

—Winston Churchill

PREFACE

Four decades ago, a young doctor — equipped with book learning and the confidence of youth — departed the nurturing cocoon of his training program ready to reach out and heal the sick and fix the wounded. His immediate expectation, devoid of much experience, was that of transactional encounters with patients: medical care in exchange for payment. He was surprised to learn that the compensation for services provided did not hold a candle to the appreciation and respect generated between patient and doctor when advocacy and trust dominated their relationship. He came to understand that meaningful connections with patients sustained his commitment to healing and aroused his desire to be the best doctor he could be.

That young man was me. I was thankful for that discovery then, and forty years later I am still in awe of the gifts derived from serving patients through patient trust and physician advocacy.

Regrettably, something changed.

A dehumanization of the way doctors serve patients poisoned the house of medicine. The importance of relationship diminished. The lifeblood of healing relationships — trust and advocacy — was pummeled.

While the cornerstones of healing traditionally involved relationship, context, compassion, and skill, the 21st-century house of medicine (with assistance from other involved stakeholders) has embraced evidence-based medicine, algorithmic order sets, electronic health records, rigid patient requirements, and physician productivity metrics.

Yes, something changed.

It's time to declare that we have all been played. Unwittingly perhaps, but nevertheless played, played to the hilt. And just as importantly it is time to ask the million-dollar question: Who has played us? Who caused patients to feel like pawns, or even worse, roadkill? Who has driven healers to quit? Who has stripped citizens of their health freedom? Who has too casually discarded the value of "informed consent"?

I will tell you who the players are — who played you, and

who played me.

I have come to recognize that medically related agendas not centered on patient wellbeing and physician guidance can be a poison to patients and doctors alike. And this is exactly the root of the problem. Schemes emanating from Big Pharma, Big Tech, and Big Government too often do not serve healers or the sick. This triad represents a dangerous and insidious force which works against transparency and health freedom. It is the triad of tyranny. Its appetite is for power, dollars, and control.

I will tell you of a new lens through which to see the forces that would do us harm.

Stories open the mind to dimensions not easily explored, and this is why I have chosen to use real-life interactions in combination with questions and topics for reflection. This book describes patient encounters with a resolute commitment to recreating authentic content. Copious notes helped me in this task, but the sheer amount of time and information involved in a patient meeting prevented a strict adherence to literal accuracy. While attempting to stay as close as possible to actual conversations, some editing was in order to avoid repetition, preserve relevance, and protect patient privacy. In situations of remarkable emotional poignancy, I amalgamated encounters to ensure preservation of anonymity for patients, families, and caregivers.

I have long believed challenges cannot be overcome without courage. This book was born of a passion to speak of the forces which fractured patient-doctor relationships, broke the house of medicine, ignored sacred oaths, and tried to cancel skeptical voices. I endeavored to hone in on the "who, what, why, when, and where" of the problems raised in these chapters, and it is alarming that virtually every concern I dissected had its birth within the realm of activity of the triad of tyranny — Big Pharma, Big Tech, and Big Government.

FOREWORD
Peter A. McCullough, MD, MPH

We will all look back on the COVID-19 years and recall certain facts or inflection points. Almost certainly we will most remember how it affected us and our families — the loss of an elderly parent or spouse, the near misses that occurred with a deceptive respiratory illness that started out as the mildest "head cold" and then weeks later was a relentless unshakable illness with brutal coughing and gasping for breath with even the slightest exertion.

We will remember the "long COVID" symptoms of brain fog, headaches, blood pressure swings, and restless sleep. Some of us would be committed to serious medications such as prolonged steroids or blood thinners. Others would suffer strokes, heart attacks, hearing loss, numbness, loss of pregnancies, and an endless array of problems after SARS-CoV-2 infection.

We would be so starved of anything to bring this onslaught to a close that when the COVID-19 vaccine programs were rolled out, we waited in line for hours and scrambled to find openings to get that needle in our arms in the early part of 2021 — anything to get some degree of protection from the fatal contagion. Little did we know that we were being "played."

How did this happen?

Ineptitude played an enormous role. Historians will ask how a handful of clinically unqualified physicians and ill-prepared agencies led a destructive pandemic response while so many of America's most credentialed and experienced doctors (who discovered and learned how to save millions of lives) were sidelined and later silenced. Over-reaching schemes by government organizations and bureaucrats became the norm, and harmful policies were enacted with anonymity and without explanation.

The insidious and progressive control over physicians and mid-level providers in the United States and all over the world was a rigid stratagem never before imposed on the medical profession.

Dr. Scott Jensen, a modern-day hero physician, legislator, and natural leader, breaks the miasma and, in a highly graphical manner, puts forward a series of tractable, irrefutable, and alarming explanations for what has happened to the way we care for one another and how the COVID-19 crisis laid bare-naked and painful truths which demonstrate that patients have become pawns on the chessboard of healthcare.

Dr. Jensen was part of a small group of doctors who realized very early on that the White House Task Force, FDA, CDC, NIH, Pharma, and the media failed to deliver updates on good news. Instead, the combined force of their messaging endlessly highlighted hospitalizations and deaths — which intensified widespread fear. A triad of tyranny — Big Pharma, Big Tech, and Big Government — unleashed ruthless powers on an unsuspecting populace, and heartbreaking collateral damage was the result. Such relentless and exquisite pain could have, and should have, been avoided.

Scott Jensen explains in a fast-moving narrative how the pieces came together to make COVID-19 crisis management a "manmade" tragedy, and he describes how this triad of tyranny has been engaging in mischievous deeds for decades. The pandemic itself was quite simply the spotlight that illuminated with dramatic clarity what had been perpetrated on patients for decades and how the healing profession had lost its way.

Only the insights and heroic actions of genuine public servants, scientists, and doctors like Scott Jensen can now save America's healthcare system. Catastrophic and unwarranted medical outcomes have already become commonplace. This brewing calamity reaches far beyond COVID-19, and Dr. Jensen explains how it is rooted in the abandonment of the most sacred vows healers make to their patients, one human to another — broken by a historical sequence of events and a series of actions and a web of contributors that is so large and interwoven it is mind-blowing.

So sit back and get ready for a fast-paced, incisive, and truly authoritative accounting of critical factors contributing to the current healthcare crisis. Dr. Jensen delivers with masterful writing, clarity of presentation, and a conviction grounded in faith, beneficence, and deep respect for each and every one of you and everything you have experienced.

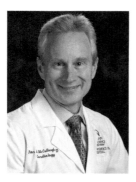

Dr. McCullough is an internist, cardiologist, and epidemiologist in Dallas, Texas, who actively manages cardiovascular complications of COVID-19 viral infections and injuries developing subsequent to COVID-19 vaccinations. Since the outset of the pandemic, Dr. McCullough has been a leader in the medical response to the COVID-19 disaster, with over fifty peer-reviewed publications related to the infection. Dr. McCullough testified to the U.S. Senate Committee on Homeland Security and Governmental Affairs and also co-moderated the U.S. Senate Panel "COVID-19: A Second Opinion," chaired by Senator Ron Johnson. He has reviewed thousands of studies and reports, participated in numerous scientific congresses and panels, and is considered one of the world's leading experts on COVID-19.

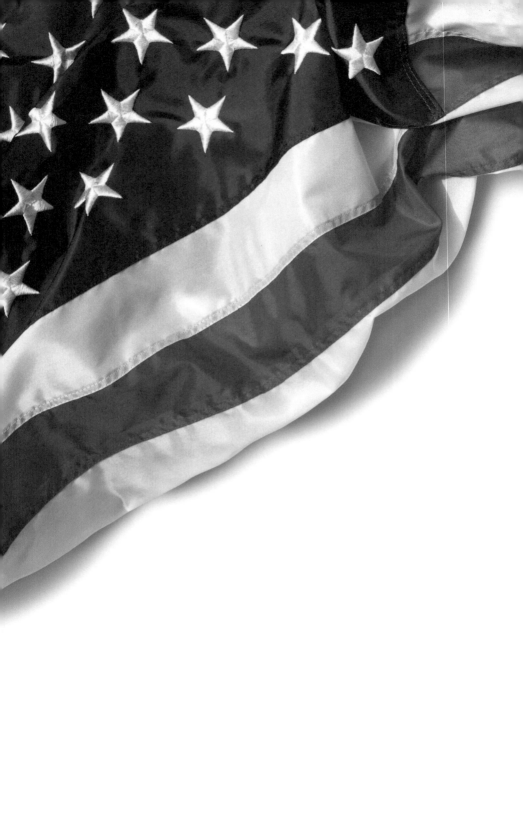

"IN A TIME OF UNIVERSAL DECEIT, TELLING THE TRUTH BECOMES A REVOLUTIONARY ACT."

—George Orwell

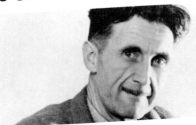

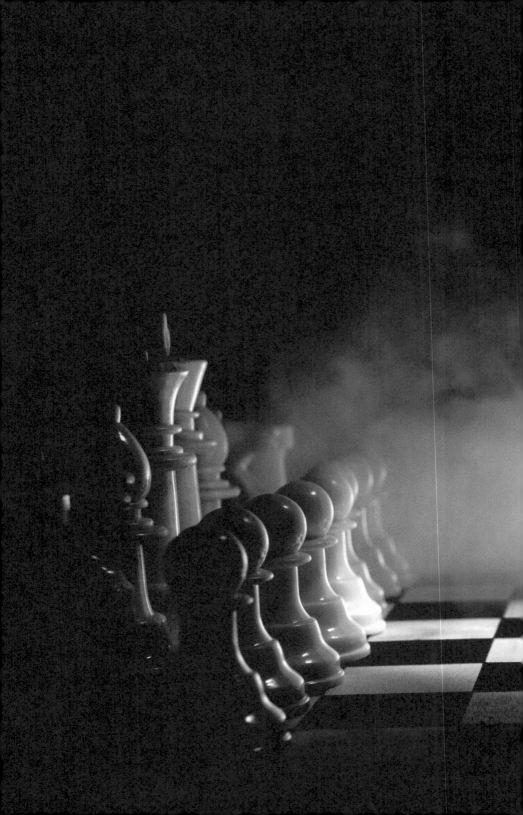

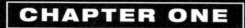

CHAPTER ONE

We've BEEN PLAYED

We've been played.

Bold statement, but true! All of us living in the United States of America have been played and are being played even now. When you fully realize what has happened in our healthcare system over the last few years, you'll recognize that we have all been conned, manipulated, and lied to — by people we thought we could trust. Yes, we have all been played, and it isn't going to stop until we stand strong and declare: ENOUGH!

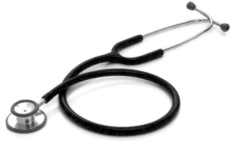

Why do I care? Why should you care? Because the cancer that for years has afflicted the U.S. healthcare system has been granted an unbelievable degree of power and control via the COVID pandemic. The malignancy killing our system of caring for one another is metastasizing in countless directions. This cancer isn't just attacking our bones and liver! It has been given free access to our hearts and minds.

And what is this cancer?

It is the relentless and malignant growth of a triad of intersecting powerbrokers: Big Pharma, Big Tech, and Big Government. This threesome of dominant societal influencers has created a new reality whereby it determines what we see, what we hear, what we discuss, and even how we live. This triumvirate is ruthlessly reshaping our lives and is every bit as deadly as any stage 4 cancer.

Its agenda is plainly visible in everyday American life and has been fueled by similar interests centering on profits, power, and control. And it is no coincidence that our world-leading healthcare system is its initial target. It can no longer be denied that a massive horizontal integration of this trio's joint interests is playing out daily. Indeed, Big Pharma, Big Tech, and Big Government have carved a path to tyrannical domination of humanity by dictating the policies which guide the world of healing and healers. That corridor of control has already expanded in a direction that is undercutting the heart of America, as its hard-working middle class bears the brunt of scientific and technological arrogance. This encroachment is a harbinger of danger for all, for when this elite triumvirate controls the masses, all our futures become subject to its self-serving tyranny.

Let it not be said that we were not forewarned.

So it has come to pass that while our healthcare system has been ill for years, the abrupt onslaught of the COVID-19 pandemic accelerated its destruction and threatens us with an almost incurable mess. Doctors bicker, politicians lie, bureaucrats fumble, and the resulting goulash is what we are left with. What may have been subtle only a few years ago has now been exposed as a monopolistic cancer dead set on dollars, power, and controlling contrarian voices.

Exposing this dangerous triad of tyranny is essential if we are to protect the fragile world in which we live. It is in sharing stories of real-life patients and real-life treacheries that the reader might begin to understand the breadth and depth of the cancer that threatens the time-honored oath professed by doctors for centuries — *primum, non nocere:* first, do no harm.

In confronting the new reality of President Dwight Eisenhower's predicted "technological and scientific elite," we must refuse to concede our health freedom without a fight. It has only been a relatively recent phenomenon — less than a century — whereby patients have been relegated to mere pawns in a trillion-dollar medical-industrial complex. Throughout the history of man, healers have served the afflicted with energy, knowledge, and advocacy. Now governments, monopolistic stakeholders, and appointed bureaucrats have found a way to gain control of the interaction between patients and doctors. Their tools include fearmongering, arrogance, and never-ending self-absorption.

But let's put a point on this discussion. Why do I care so much? Why do I put myself in ridicule's way by challenging the

U.S. healthcare dysfunction?

Because with every fiber in my being I believe the intersection of a broken house of medicine, a power-driven corrupt government, and the growing incestuous relationship between Big Pharma, Big Tech, and Big Government is taking America to a place far darker than we have ever known. This is a place in need of illumination by the bright lights of transparency and hope, so that a piercing discussion regarding informed consent, health freedom, and immoral policies can take place in the public square. In short, we must begin to view the world through a new lens that sharpens our focus on a menacing triad which exercises control through tyranny.

We stand at a crossroads in time, and this book may be nothing more than a small step on the way to rediscovering the wisdom of our Founding Fathers when they bequeathed to us their ultimate gift — freedom. But a small step is, nonetheless, a step.

Let's begin our discussion with a story about a patient.

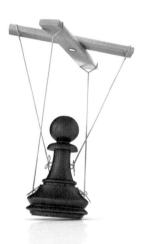

We must begin to view the world through a new lens that sharpens our focus on a menacing triad which exercises control through tyranny.

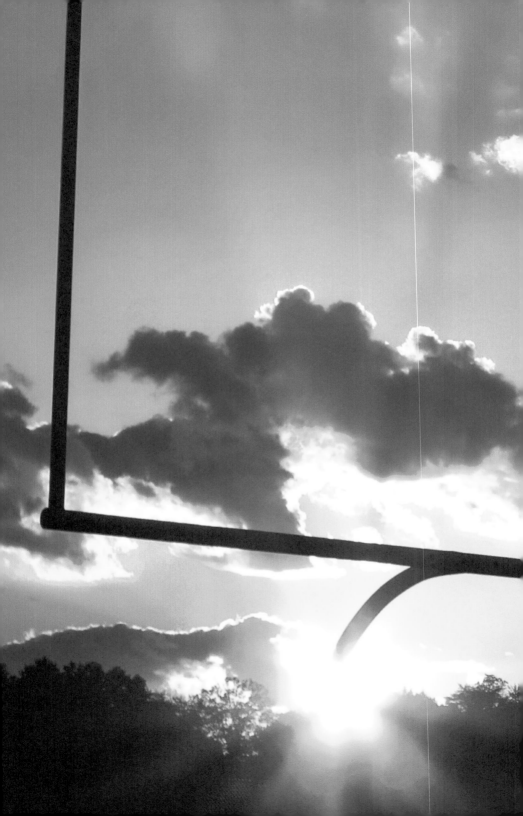

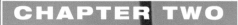

CHAPTER TWO

MOVING THE
GOALPOSTS

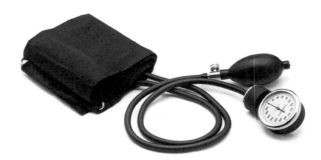

When patients first came to me at the beginning of the COVID-19 pandemic, they were scared. They wanted to do their part and they wanted science-based information. I shared what I knew, leaning heavily on what was coming from the White House task force, specifically Dr. Fauci and Dr. Birx.

After a month or so my patients seemed relieved that no existential crisis of the human race was at hand and were ready for their lives to return to normal. It didn't happen. Even though the twin pillars of "flatten the curve" and "prevent overload of healthcare facilities" had apparently been achieved, the lockdown continued. Then my patients grew angry. The goalposts had been moved, without any transparent scientific explanation. Flawed modeling programs were determinants for rapidly created policies by state governors. Bureaucratic authority grew, individual liberties shrank, and business owners no longer had the freedom to decide if they would be open or closed or what hours they would serve their customers.

Lockdowns did not end. They were extended — indefinitely. And what happened next should have been foreseen: public trust disintegrated.

Doctors would do well to learn from this event, because patients often view doctors as moving the goalposts of targeted therapies. Let me give you an example.

* * *

A few years back a patient came in to see me. You've probably met the kind of man I'm writing about. He's the type who carries his own sunshine with him wherever he goes. But not today. I immediately noticed that Bill was not his usual happy-go-lucky self, but looked perplexed. After we exchanged our usual pleasantries, my typically upbeat patient said in a subdued tone, "Doc, what's going on here?"

I responded, "What do you mean, Bill?"

"Doc, you told me a couple years ago that I needed to lower my LDL cholesterol from 180 to less than 130. So I started to take Lipitor to do that, and it worked, right?"

He was 100 percent correct and had needed the maximum dose of Lipitor to achieve success.

"That's right, and your last LDL was 120."

"Then why did my cardiologist tell me a couple months ago that I had a problem and needed to take another pill to lower my LDL to less than 100?"

Alarm bells went off in my head when I heard him say that. I felt for him. I knew why he was confused, and I would have felt confused as well. So I leaned back and told him the truth about doctors and pills and researchers and drug companies.

"Bill, what's happening is that doctors, medical researchers, and pharmaceutical companies often work hand-in-hand in terms of research being done and recommendations made. For example, if a study is done which concludes that patients with diabetes should get their LDL to less than 100 to lower their theoretical risk for heart attack, then cardiology associations usually recommend that doctors work with their patients to reach the target number. It gets arbitrary and sometimes even silly. So here's the problem. Recently you were diagnosed with diabetes. Before you had diabetes an LDL upper limit of 130 LDL was fine. But once you got labeled with diabetes, things changed, and the recommended LDL upper limit became 100."

Bill's eyes widened and he said, "C'mon, Doc, I feel like I'm chasing my tail. You know as well as I do that I didn't even have diabetes UNTIL I started taking the Lipitor to get my LDL under 130. And I didn't even know I had high cholesterol until I came in for my physical. I should never have listened to my wife about needing a checkup. And now, what the heck! I actually think the diabetes was caused by the Lipitor, and now I've got a specialist telling me I have to lower my cholesterol even more with more pills. Why don't we just stop the Lipitor and see if the diabetes goes away! You remember how upset I was when you told me I had diabetes last year. This is crazy. One thing leads to another, and everything leads to more pills. You get where I'm coming from, Doc? Maybe I should just take my chances with high cholesterol?"

"Bill, I understand. It's immensely frustrating. Most doctors don't tell their patients that if they go on Lipitor they are potentially increasing their odds of developing type II diabetes.

And most doctors certainly aren't going to tell you that if you develop diabetes in response to Lipitor, the recommendation would be the commonsense approach of dropping the Lipitor. Instead, they're going to recommend increasing it. As weird as that sounds, it's the truth. It's a perfect example of moving the goalposts on the patient. I don't blame you at all if you don't buy into what you're being told. If I were in your situation I would struggle as well. Frankly, if I were in your shoes, I would want to stop the Lipitor and see if my blood sugars return to normal non-diabetic levels. If they do I would really go after my cholesterol with aggressive lifestyle changes. By that I mean a better diet, fewer carbohydrates, more exercise, lose 20 pounds, do some muscle strengthening, stretch every day, and increase the fiber in your diet. And by the way, I do think cutting back on the beer would help."

Bill looked at me long and hard, and finally said, "Okay, Doc, I get it. I'm at a crossroads. I'm sticking with you. I'm not interested in seeing the cardiologist again and I am just not buying what he's selling. And I don't appreciate him moving the darn goalposts."

I hesitated a bit and then said, "Bill, let's stop the Lipitor. We'll do a baseline check today on your LDL, and then we'll check it again in two months along with a fasting sugar and an A1c to evaluate your diabetes. In the meantime, let's get serious on those lifestyle changes."

He grinned and seemed more like his usual self. "I understand, Doc. Thanks. I appreciate you."

As he walked down the hallway, I smiled at the privilege of being a family doctor.

* * *

Here's the takeaway that we need to be aware of going forward. Due to the increased involvement of pharmaceutical companies in funding medical studies and the desire for researchers to secure solid funding sources for their projects, we increasingly see the "goalposts" moved because research outcomes can often be interpreted in such a way as to support more pills. And you won't see many studies designed to reduce the number of pills used by patients. So if doctors and patients want to cut down on pills, they're on their own, and doctors may be putting themselves at risk of ridicule or discipline from colleagues, professional associations, and insurance companies. Sometimes even malpractice cases will be spawned by an adverse outcome resulting from the discontinuation of medicines. Doctors are not enthusiastic about cutting back on pills because the *status quo* is safer. Reducing pills takes a lot of time during an office visit because of the necessary discussion involved with making changes. A lot of doctors would rather keep you on a program of medications and simply see you in three months to check on how you are doing.

Standard blood pressure recommendations are another example of moving goalposts. If scientific studies conclude that target systolic blood pressure values should be lowered from 150 to 140, a lot more patients will need blood pressure pills. This is a tried and tested way for pharmaceutical companies to sell more medications and increase profits. Then, if taking more blood pressure pills causes more problems — such as erectile dysfunction — then there will be a lot of guys interested in Viagra and more pills will be taken. The cycle of Big Pharma funding medical research which determines that more pills are necessary predictably results in more pills consumed by patients.

Is it any surprise that no country on the planet takes more prescription drugs than the United States of America? And by the way, we pay a higher price tag than any other country as well.

You get my point? Patients need to champion their own health and may need to make decisions in opposition to physician recommendations. And patients may need to declare, "No more moving the goalposts!" Doctors don't always get it right, and that is why I remind my patients that doctors *practice* medicine.

After four decades of caring for patients, I have learned an important lesson: Today's science may be tomorrow's folly — but that won't stop doctors from being overly confident that the prescriptions they write are the "absolute best medicine" for their patients.

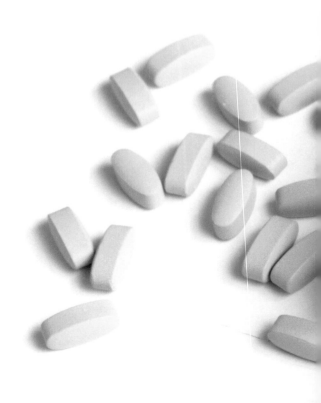

CHAPTER THREE

FOLLOW THE
MONEY

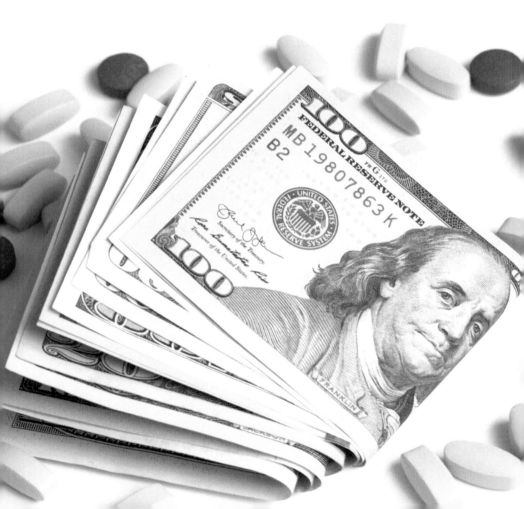

Charlie was frowning when I walked into the exam room.

"What's up, Charlie?" I asked. "Where's your usual smile?"

Charlie began by telling me, "Doc, this whole COVID nightmare has had me on edge for more than a year. I couldn't get to the gym and with the winter and holidays, I put on 20 pounds, and now I have high blood pressure."

"Were you told that by another doctor?" I asked.

"What do you mean?" he responded. "You're my doctor."

"Exactly," I said. "The reason I asked is because I don't remember diagnosing you with hypertension. So where did you get the idea that you have high blood pressure?"

"Well, Doc, Amy and I started subscribing to a new health magazine, and they had a big article in it, and according to what we read, I have high blood pressure."

I chuckled, got out the blood pressure cuff, and said, "Okay, you know the drill." Charlie immediately began rolling up his right sleeve. I put the cuff on him and his blood pressure was 140/88.

"Your blood pressure is fine, Charlie, and if you lighten up a little and relax a bit, it'll probably drop a few points once we finish the physical and get the prostate check done."

And as a matter of fact it did. Fifteen minutes after his first measurement, his next reading was 136/82.

"Charlie," I said, "I don't want you to be overly alarmed when your blood pressure jumps around some. That's pretty typical. You might be surprised at how much anxiety can elevate your blood pressure. What you said at the beginning of our appointment about gaining 20 pounds and not getting to the gym has a *powerful influence on your blood pressure."*

I continued: "Here's something else I want you to appreciate. When I began my medical career in 1978, a blood pressure reading of 160/90 was considered acceptable in many settings. But since then I have seen the recommended values repeatedly get adjusted. The recommendation for the upper number, the systolic pressure, has changed from 160 to 150, from 150 to 140, and then to 135, and even 130. Now it has swung back again so that 150 can be acceptable for folks above the age of 65. My point is that science has not been able to establish with certainty what an ideal blood pressure reading should be. Granted, it would have been nice had our Creator given us an owner's manual at birth telling us exactly what is a normal blood pressure, but that's not how it works."

Charlie, looked puzzled and asked, "Doc, why do they keep changing the numbers?"

I had his attention. "Take a guess, Charlie."

He laughed loudly and said, "Follow the money! Drug companies!"

"You got it. Big Pharma has a powerful influence on medical standards. In fact, they have one of the largest groups of lobbyists in Washington, D.C., and they know how to throw their weight around. The number of dollars politicians get from pharmaceutical companies is obscene. Their dollars talk — and not just with politicians.

"Big Pharma knows that we have an epidemic of obesity in the U.S. today with more than 67 percent of all adults falling into the overweight or obese category. Obesity can elevate blood pressure and cholesterol. So what does Big Pharma do? They strategically

fund research studies which are likely to conclude that lowering blood pressure and cholesterol improves health. The potential dangers of pills, pills, and more pills are usually minimized, and doctors read the study results and prescribe more pills."

It was clear I had Charlie's undivided attention, so I went on: "Let's say that you are a medical research scientist and you want funding for your next project. You have to find the dollars to pay for the study and its expenses — chemicals, equipment, personnel, etc. If a pharmaceutical company funds the research, where do you think that scientist might look to get his next study financed? Would he not look to the same source as had supported his previous research? And wouldn't the pharmaceutical company be more likely to fund studies that reach the conclusion that more aggressive use of medications would decrease cholesterol or blood pressure and maybe save lives?

"So Charlie, you see the cycle I am talking about. Studies recommending more drugs lead to more available funding which might lead to more studies concluding that more drugs are better. It's a vicious circle and we can see how pharmaceutical companies might fund study after study if they like the results. And it is interesting to note that these results are not always reproduced in other first-world countries. We need to be more than a little skeptical when considering some of these studies."

Charlie nodded and said, "Wow, Doc, I had no idea! I just need to 'follow the money' to understand more about the medical field."

When he left the exam room, it was my hope that Charlie would be less anxious about his blood pressure and more skeptical about more pills.

* * *

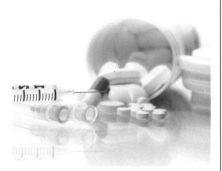

How do we hold the pharmaceutical industry accountable, knowing that drug companies are on the lookout for the next billion-dollar block-buster drug?

On July 12, 2004, it was announced that the standard reading for "acceptable" LDL cholesterol for many patients (with certain diagnoses) should be revised from 130 to less than 100. In other words, overnight the new healthy standard had dropped by 30 points. Why? Because studies had revealed a statistically significant benefit. These statistics can be massaged easily, so I frequently advise patients to spend some time "Googling" the concept of NNT (number needed to treat — a practical statistical indicator helping patients understand the actual likelihood of benefit for them). When studies call for more pills, Big Pharma can make billions almost overnight because thousands of patients might be prescribed the medicines involved with the research.

When research drives the standard threshold for high blood pressure from 140/90 mm Hg to a new threshold of 135/85 mm Hg, the end result may be millions of new prescriptions written to lower blood pressure. But at what risk to patients? Side effects of blood pressure medications are numerous, and serious complications include dizziness, lightheadedness, and falls associated with hip fractures and brain bleeds.

Here are a few questions to ponder: How do we address the situation that now exists with pharmaceutical companies funding ever more medical studies because researchers need funding sources?

Does the fact that universities require faculty members to accomplish a certain number of research projects in order to obtain tenure aggravate the overall problem?

How can doctors make certain that experimental results represent good reproducible science worthy of changing patient recommendations utilized in everyday medical care? Do patients become mere pawns in this dollar-driven industry in which more pills consumed correlates with greater profits? Does a patient taking more than a dozen pills a day represent a target goal for Big Pharma?

Do desired research outcomes have too much impact on the actual final conclusions of studies? How do we hold the pharmaceutical industry accountable, knowing that drug companies are on the lookout for the next billion-dollar blockbuster drug?

How do we balance the best interests of the American people with the expensive discoveries brought forth by the pharmaceutical industry? What regulatory measures can be set in place to reduce abuses and yet protect the culture of hard-driving exploration and creativity which can translate into game-changing cures for humans?

Is there any motivation for Big Pharma to participate in the quest to fix a broken and expensive healthcare system, so that patient needs once more become the primary consideration? Or is Big Pharma only interested in continuously expanding the size of the country's healthcare budget and appetite for drugs?

How does government policy get reshaped to rein in the corporate thirst to ride fast, hard, and as long as possible on the U. S. healthcare gravy train?

"NO ONE SHOULD APPROACH THE TEMPLE OF SCIENCE WITH THE SOUL OF A MONEY CHANGER."

—Thomas Browne

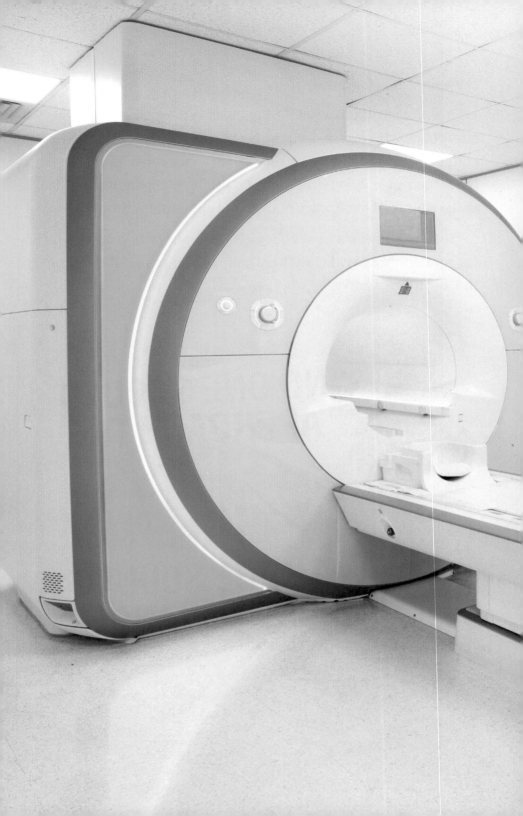

CHAPTER FOUR

THE BROKEN HOUSE OF MEDICINE

It had been a long but good day, and I decided to stop for dinner at a favorite restaurant on my way home. As I was waiting for my food to arrive, a friend I hadn't seen in some time walked over to say hello. Jim told me about his family and what everyone was up to and I told him about mine. Abruptly his voice took on a serious tone, "Doc, can I ask you a question?"

I nodded, "Sure."

He then said, "I've been seeing the same doctor for a long time, but a few days ago he told me that I would have to find a new doctor because he was retiring. I was shocked. He can't be much older than 50, so I asked him why. He just shrugged and said something about wanting to consider different options. Truth is, Doc, it was obvious he didn't want to talk about it, but I don't think he was being up front with me. So I'm curious, why would a physician that young be throwing in the towel? He's got years of medical practice ahead of him. He worked his tail off to become a doctor. Can you tell me what's really happening? Why are doctors that young retiring and leaving their patients?"

I took a deep breath and pushed my chair back a bit. "Okay, Jim, have a seat. This may take a while."

He sat and I talked.

"I'm not your doctor, you're not my patient, and I'll just shoot straight from the hip. Being a doctor has changed a lot since I went to medical school. Frankly, Jim, what you are seeing is the broken house of medicine. My profession is fractured. Nowadays, there are intense pressures that doctors live with in caring for patients. Most people can't imagine the frustration that many physicians experience in everyday practice. Their autonomy has been taken

away and administrative protocols disrupt their ability to develop relationships with their patients. The time it takes to document the essentials of a patient visit has grown, and the joy in caring for patients too often is gone. On top of that, physicians often feel they can't do what is in a patient's best interest because of the drive to reduce expenditures. This isn't just annoying, but downright humiliating, especially when a doctor knows exactly what needs to be done. Too often we're just not allowed to do it."

After a pause to gather my thoughts I forged ahead: "I'm sure you've heard about the risk of malpractice and that certainly is problematic, but actually, that's usually not the big issue. When I talk to my colleagues I hear about rigid rules, departmental regulations, and insurance guidelines. When doctors are pushed to make sure they are producing enough revenue and advised that they are not seeing enough patients to hit their production targets, that's tough on them. Doctors don't think of their patients as units, and don't appreciate being interrupted by staff because a patient's allotted time is up. Some patient visits take a little longer than others, and it breaks my heart to see doctors reading articles on how to keep long-winded patients off their schedules.

"It has also become increasingly common for physicians to be informed mid-year by insurance companies that they have to change a patient's medicines simply because the insurance company changed their formulary (menu) of drugs available for patients. (This requirement for substitution may result from a lower bid for a similar drug from a competing pharmaceutical company, which sets in motion a process of exchanging different pills for a patient and the physician is responsible for approving such medication changes.) Honestly Jim, we are being pitted

against the very patients who rely on us to advocate for them. It's gotten crazy and a lot of doctors are just saying, 'The hell with it.'

"Take, for example, the patient who comes to the clinic in obvious pain and can barely move. The physician asks what the problem is, and the patient describes a low back pain that is so debilitating he can't get comfortable either sitting or standing, and can't sleep at night. One thing physicians consider in such situations is to schedule an MRI to determine the source of the problem, and yet they may not be allowed to do so because of insurance company guidelines declaring that the patient has to experience symptoms for at least six weeks before an MRI will be covered. Of course, that's insane. Physicians are by nature compassionate, which is why most of them became doctors to begin with. They want to alleviate human suffering. And now they're being prevented from doing so.

"Or how about this one? I have a friend, Brad, who has a granddaughter that is a year-and-a-half old. Her parents can't find her a doctor because their concerns about potential adverse effects of vaccines is something physicians don't want to deal with. Physicians may be hesitant to get involved with such a family because of the need for lengthy discussions and the fact that doctors are being monitored by administrators, insurance companies, and public health departments for vaccination rates. Some clinics grade doctor performance based on how many kids don't complete the routine schedule of vaccinations, and this can even impact what kind of bonus dollars a doctor might be eligible for at the end of the year. Don't kid yourself, Jim, this is tough on doctors. We hate many of these guidelines, but can't do anything about them. And it frustrates us to no end.

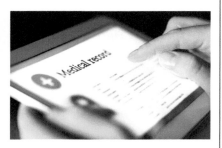

The joy of practicing medicine, the privilege of caring for patients, and the passion to truly be "healers" must be reawakened in doctors if we are going to see the quality of medical care turned around.

"When I first went into medicine it wasn't like that. I made the best possible judgment calls on behalf of my patients and so did my colleagues. Nowadays, more and more of my colleagues that work in hospital clinics are relegated to the dictates of insurance companies and Big Pharma working together. They want to help their patients to the very best of their ability, but they feel as though their hands are tied, and they are not being allowed to help patients in the most effective and humane ways possible.

"Additionally, Jim, there are doctors who are actually ridiculed for the way they care for their patients. Our profession is indeed fractured, and COVID-19 has made it far worse. I'll tell you honestly, I have had doctors who have never met me that have gone on social media saying that I should not be allowed to practice medicine. Why? Who knows? Was it because they don't think patients should have access to drugs like hydroxychloroquine or ivermectin, but I'm willing to prescribe them? I tell you, Jim, caring for patients has gotten more and

more difficult, and common sense has become uncommon.

"Younger physicians went into medicine thinking that it would be more satisfying than it is, while older physicians look at younger physicians and wonder why they are so willing to plug a patient into an algorithm rather than explain things and find out where the patient is with the various treatment options. The frustration patients have with what they perceive to be a cookie cutter mentality by doctors is understandable, but the truth is that many doctors believe they have no power to change a one-size-fits-all approach.

"So, my very long answer to your question is that I think most doctors are independent, highly motivated individuals. It took intelligence, perseverance, and hard work for them to become doctors. American medicine is at a crossroad and many doctors don't really know who they are working for. They wonder if they are working for insurance companies to keep utilization costs down. Or are they working for Big Pharma and are no longer able to prescribe highly effective generic drugs that cost only a fraction of their brand-name counterpart? Or maybe they're working for a combined hospital and clinic entity called an "accountable care organization," which is often governed by the edict: 'We set the rules and at the end of the year, if you do a good job of holding costs down, you'll get a bonus check, and if you don't do a good job of keeping costs down, your pay will be docked.' The bottom line is that the notion of doctors serving patients is becoming increasingly old-fashioned and out of vogue.

"So Jim, I guess it's really no surprise that there are more and more doctors who are so frustrated that they are calling it quits."

After a moment of silence, Jim responded thoughtfully: "I guess

I got more than I asked for, Doc. Thanks, I guess." He got up and returned to his cold hamburger and warm beer.

* * *

Here are a few critical questions that help to reveal the extent of the brokenness within the U.S. healthcare system:

How does the broken house of medicine heal from within?

How can the joy of medicine and privilege of caring for patients be reawakened in doctors when the hassles of electronic health records, productivity expectations, financial stresses, insurance rules and regulations, informed consent requirements, malpractice fears, government intrusions, documentation standards, and unrealistic patient expectations all combine to erode career satisfaction and destroy the revitalizing nature of a healthy patient-doctor relationship?

How does the patient once again become the focus of our healthcare system, rather than a pawn in a convoluted bureaucracy filled with dollar-driven stakeholders?

How do we repair the relationship between the healer and the sick?

How can insurance companies and Big Pharma do what they need to do without the almighty dollar corrupting the essence of caring for the sick, the wounded, and the hurting?

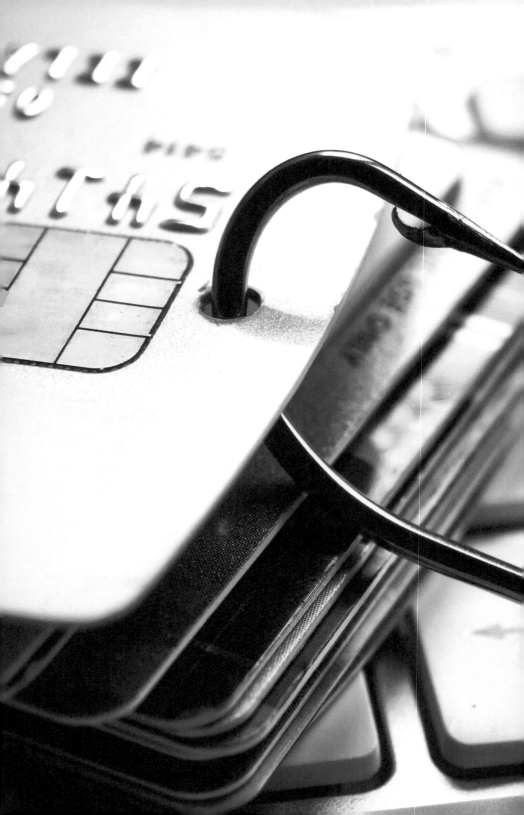

CHAPTER FIVE

PAID FOR BY
WHOM?

It has been fascinating for me to reflect on the types of people I meet as a family doctor. I have found it particularly interesting to learn about the tolerance for pain folks exhibit. At one end of the spectrum are patients who can endure a massive amount of pain, but on the other side of the continuum I have encountered people who cry uncontrollably because they bumped their knee on a coffee table. The man I'm about to discuss had an immense ability to withstand discomfort. He epitomizes the word, "stoic," which is defined by Merriam-Webster's Dictionary as "someone apparently indifferent to pleasure or pain."

* * *

We all know guys like Pete, the kind of man who can pull a metal sliver from the center of his palm without even wincing. So when I opened the exam room door and saw Pete, I knew that something serious was amiss or he wouldn't be there.

Unfortunately, I was right. A simple glance told me he was in a world of hurt. He could hardly move. I empathized with him instantly and wanted to help in any way possible.

I asked him, "What's happening, Pete? It's obvious you're hurting."

He responded, "I'm not sure what I did, Doc. I was working on my dock and I bent over to prop it up with a piece of wood and all of a sudden I felt a sharp twinge. I could hardly stand up. I don't know quite what I did. I always figured I was in good enough shape that this wouldn't happen to me. But the fact is, I'm moving like an old man, I can't sleep at night, and the pain is pretty bad."

"When did this happen, Pete?"

He said, "A couple weeks ago. I thought it'd get better if I just took it easy, but it's only gotten worse. I've done the icing and I've taken Tylenol and Advil, but nothing seems to help."

"Well, you've done the right things, but obviously, there's still a problem."

"Yeah, Doc, it's getting worse every day. I had no idea how bad something like this could really be. What should I do? Get an MRI or something? What do you think?"

"I need a little more information, Pete. Does the pain radiate at all? Does it run down your legs or up into your neck?"

"No, nothing like that, Doc. I just feel it in my back on the right side just above my pelvis."

I examined him as best I could and then said, "Pete, I want to do an x-ray and then maybe get you into physical therapy."

"Okay, Doc, I'm fine with the x-ray, and I can do some more ibuprofen, but there is no way I could do physical therapy. At least not right now. I can barely move."

I then said, "Well, we may want to try some steroids."

Pete looked at me quizzically and said, "Steroids? I don't know if that's what I want to do."

"Well, Pete, let's hold tight for a bit until I get a chance to look at your x-rays."

Twenty minutes later I told him, "Pete your x-rays look okay. There's no fracture, but there is evidence of muscle spasm. Let's try a regimen of low-dose steroids along with ibuprofen, keep the ice going, and hopefully you will feel better soon so we can start some physical therapy."

There was a long pause and Pete said, "Can't we just get an MRI? My brother had something like this happen a couple of years ago, and after he suffered for about two weeks his doctor scheduled an MRI which showed a ruptured disc. It would be nice to know what I'm dealing with."

I hesitated and said, "I'm sorry, Pete, but with your insurance, you have to have symptoms for six weeks before they'll pay for it. Your insurance company needs to authorize the MRI in order for them to pay for it. Pete, it's sort of like your homeowner's insurance when you have to first get approval from the insurance company to replace a storm-damaged roof, because if you don't, then you pay for the new roof."

"What?" Pete blurted. "Are you kidding me, Doc? I've been paying insurance for years and never used it. Now I got a problem and you're telling me I have to wait six weeks to find out what's going on? That's crazy!"

I said, "Pete, that's the situation with your insurance company. I'm sorry, but I don't make the rules. It is what it is."

"Well how much would it cost if I just paid for it myself?" he asked.

"It would probably be around three grand," I said. "Look, Pete, MRIs are expensive and if we do one I don't want you to have to pay for it. The x-ray doesn't show much, and as I already mentioned, steroids and ibuprofen might help a lot. I promise you that if we need the MRI in another four weeks, we will get the authorization from the insurance company if I have to call them myself. I'm sorry for the hassle and delay, but when it comes to expensive tests and insurance companies, a key question is always, *'paid for by whom?'"*

(What Pete didn't know was that I, unfortunately, often had to spend thirty to sixty minutes arguing with an authorizing doctor from another country as to why I need to get an MRI on my patient. Pete was already riled enough.)

"Unbelievable!" he muttered. "Okay, Doc, give me the steroids."

He left and was understandably very disappointed.

* * *

Unfortunately, Pete's situation is a common one these days because the "payor" is frequently an insurance company or a government program that has specific guidelines in place restricting a physician's options. Patients are astonished to learn that what their doctor thinks is the best plan isn't necessarily going to determine what happens. It's a brutal lesson, and often provokes the patient to ask, "Who are you working for, Doc?"

Here are some questions worth asking:

How can our healthcare system balance the wants and needs of patients with the rules of insurance companies?

Should the payor be able to establish rigid rules which govern a patient's care?

Should the insurance company be required to pay for something it has determined is not necessary?

How should the patient be involved in paying for procedures not regarded as necessary by the insurance company?

These are the questions which can give shape to potential solutions. Regardless, our system of caring for patients is fragmented and shrouded by underhanded rules, excessive regulations, convoluted contract language, and hidden agendas. Pete's story puts a bright light on the serious problem of having a plan of care put together by a patient and doctor only to see it ignored by the insurance company.

Our system of caring cannot allow patients to be treated like pawns in a game of cost control and delay tactics. Insurance policies should not dictate your healthcare management, and yet they do. This tension rightfully riles many patients because nothing is more important than their health. Patients "play with fire" when they allow insurance companies to dictate what they can have done in terms of healthcare services.

But on the other hand, what a patient sees as a "need" may actually represent merely a "want," and an insurance company cannot be expected to pay for everything on a patient's wish list.

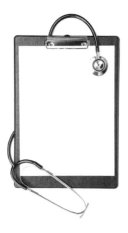

"It is better to be divided by truth than to be united in error. It is better to speak the truth that hurts and then heals, than falsehood that comforts and then kills. It is better to be hated for telling the truth than to be loved for telling a lie. It is better to stand alone with the truth, than to be wrong with a multitude. It is better to ultimately succeed with the truth than to temporarily succeed with a lie."

—Adrian Rogers

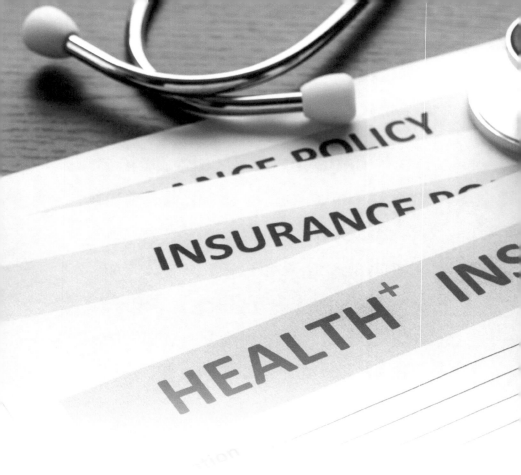

CHAPTER SIX

THE MORAL HAZARD OF A SAFETY NET

It should come as no surprise to anyone that our broken healthcare system is, in large part, due to escalating costs, inflated utilization of services, too many low-value services, the growing use of medication, and extravagant end-of-life expenses. These factors raise the ever-present question: who should pay?

But we have another deeper fundamental issue to confront: Why do we have insurance, and what are we hoping to accomplish with it?

Health insurance can be described as a collective effort to defray or reduce the impact of large or unexpected bills resulting from utilization of healthcare services. It is structured through the recruitment of a significant number of individuals who collectively see value in making advance payments to a fund which would be available to support them if they experienced an "eligible need." Their advance payments primarily serve to cushion against unplanned bills and would generally apply to health emergencies or costly procedures that could — in the moment — critically disrupt a person's financial stability. The fear of such a predicament is real and highly motivating for insurance acquisition. Thus, it can be said that the collective effort of numerous people mutually paying into a fund for protection against unanticipated financial woes is well-intentioned.

But is health insurance doing what we want, or is it disincentivizing appropriate choices? Is insurance coverage allowing people to adopt a "no skin in the game" attitude so that foolish and dangerous decisions may be more acceptable because "my health insurance will take care of things"? Does this safety net represent a moral hazard by reducing the incentive for individuals to utilize traditional moral guidance to guard against risk? Does protecting people from the consequences of their decisions generate a hazard for their health in an immoral manner? When consequential decisions are made cavalierly and without concern for potential adverse outcomes because of the existence of insurance or any other safety net, is the hazard to one's health the only consideration? How does the lack of incentive to guard oneself against risk impact the long-term solvency of the American healthcare system?

All of these are important questions. The very purpose for which insurance is created can be undermined by the very security it provides. What do I mean? I am referring to the previously discussed notion of a "moral hazard" which occurs when insurance designed to protect an individual from financial harm also creates an unintended lack of incentive to guard against unnecessary risks because that individual feels protected against the consequences of hazardous decisions he or she might make. Thus, if an individual senses he or she will have no further financial responsibility beyond the payments to the collective insurance fund, making wise and safe decisions may seem less important. In this scenario, dangerous acts of commission or omission may become more acceptable since financial considerations are no longer problematic.

In other words, if someone has the security associated with a safety net of insurance, he or she may more willingly dismiss the natural motivation for proactively safeguarding his or her personal health. That is to say, "Don't worry, if a problem develops, insurance will take care of it." Bicycle or motorcycle helmets may be scoffed at. Seat belts may be ignored. Diving off a waterfall may seem worth trying. And of greatest importance, the risks of obesity, tobacco use, and harmful lifestyle choices will be less financially consequential and therefore possibly more acceptable to those whose health is blessed by youth and a lack of chronic diseases.

Here's an example of how a mindset comforted by having insurance coverage did not necessarily encourage a person to become healthy.

* * *

I had a patient named Sally, who I thoroughly enjoyed, but despite all of our conversations about her health and the changes she could make to improve her overall well-being, she made no changes. The truth is, while she was curious to know more about how lifestyle choices impact long-term health, she seemed, deep down, to care little about how her health picture might evolve. She ignored my encouragements that she, ultimately, was the champion of her own health and that there were numerous steps she could take to enhance her downstream years. Oh sure, she gave lip service to my words, but did virtually nothing other than engage in never-ending conversations during office visits about the wonderful potential of this or that article she read about in a health prevention magazine. But when push came to shove, even though I had specifically identified one particular lifestyle change that could potentially make all the difference in the world for her foundational health, she did not make any changes.

Finally, an encounter of inevitable gentle confrontation arrived, and I pointedly asked several tough questions to promote personal accountability. She deflected them all, causing me to ask myself, "Why isn't she willing to follow through and make a change?"

The answer was simple, but not what I expected. Sally thought briefly on my questions and then confessed rather bluntly, "Dr. Jensen, I'm sorry I frustrate you. You've been clear on the value of the suggested changes I could make and the potential benefits to my health they might bring. Your instructions have been straightforward, but I must tell you, making those changes is just too hard. For your suggestions to have any real value, these lifestyle adjustments would have to be permanent. That would intrude on the way I like to live my life. This may be difficult for you to understand, but frankly, I have good health insurance that I pay for myself. If anything really does go wrong, you will be here to take care of me, and the insurance company will cover the bill for whatever is needed. Whether right or wrong, that provides me a very real measure of comfort, and relying on you and my insurance is a lot simpler than making frustrating changes in the way I live my life, which by the way could end up being a waste of time and a source of anxiety for me. You could probably say I am too complacent. Maybe I am. But living my way suits me fine because I trust that you and the insurance coverage provide a real safety net for me. That makes me feel secure. I wish I could be stronger, but at least I have you as a good fallback if I need it."

* * *

I could not help but feel touched by Sally's sincerity and her trust in me, but at the same time, her willingness to depend on me and her insurance policy was disconcerting. I had never considered that I could be a part of the problem and that by providing compassionate care for my patients, I might enable a misguided sense of security that would make pursuing optimal health less likely. I wanted to blame the insurance company, but I knew I had to own a part of the fact that Sally's moral hazard was born of both her insurance and her doctor.

Unfortunately, no matter how great your insurance policy is, insurance cannot make you healthy. Nor can your doctor. But somehow the existence of moral hazards has to be addressed, because they very much contribute to the brokenness of our healthcare system.

It is unfortunate that the peace of mind derived by an insurance policy could cause a patient to not avoid future devastation. But on the other hand, it is unrealistic to think that a return to a cash system of payment for all healthcare services is feasible. The security of insurance is vital for millions of people around the globe, and it will exist in one form or another for a long time to come.

And it makes no sense for doctors to strive for anything less than a supportive and trust-based relationship with patients.

So here we are. Patients may be lulled into a false sense of security created by insurance and caring doctors, but ultimately they will have to face the consequences of their poor health choices. They may not realize the toll their decisions will impose on themselves or the healthcare system, or the consequences to family members. I am convinced that the open discussion of moral hazards can help expose the unintended and perverse consequences of good intentions, and hopefully spur new perspectives which might actually create incentives for individuals to pursue healthy lifestyles regardless of insurance coverage.

Here are some questions to ponder:

To what extent do moral hazards undermine a healthcare system's potential for achieving the mission of providing basic healthcare for all?

How do we create a structure in which moral hazards do not create dilemmas for patients' future health?

How can insurance companies devise incentives for those they insure to actively make healthy decisions?

How can physicians effectively encourage patients to get healthier without unfairly judging them? How can the difficult conversations regarding inactivity, obesity, and alcohol abuse be optimized to affect change without sabotaging the patient-doctor relationship?

How does society ask patients to share in the real costs of poor decisions without being less than compassionate?

How do patients and physicians mutually and respectfully combine efforts to decrease the burden placed on the healthcare system by those who make poor personal health decisions?

How do doctors participate best in persuading people like Sally that their future will be healthier and happier if they will make the challenging choices necessary to optimize the well-being of mind, body, and soul?

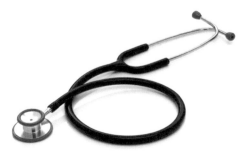

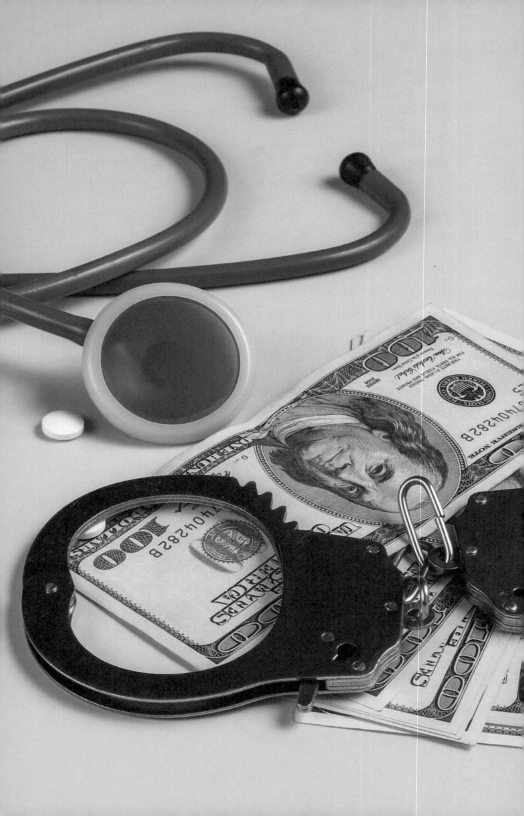

CHAPTER SEVEN

GOUGING
THE
MARKETPLACE

"Dr. Scott, do you get frustrated with the world of pills?"

I was taken aback by the question, partly because of who was asking it, a young woman named Jennifer, who happens to be a pharmacist. She is also one of my patients. I couldn't help but shake my head and laugh a little.

"Okay," I said. "Before I answer, please tell me why you're asking?"

She smiled and said, "That's fair enough," and then went on to say, "You know, Dr. Jensen, I chose to become a pharmacist because I thought I could help a lot of people make healthier choices. But frankly, I have become more and more disillusioned and skeptical by what I see happening."

"Oh, really? And what is that?" I asked.

"Here's an example," she said. "I noticed for the past several months that there is a new drug that has taken off like a rocket and is now replacing Lipitor as the most commonly prescribed statin. The advertising for the new replacement drug is off the charts. Yet, there is no real proof or evidence that it is any more effective than Lipitor, which has been the single best selling drug in history. I'm sure that you are well aware that atorvastatin, which is the generic form of Lipitor, is now only a fraction of the price that Lipitor once was and it is every bit as effective as Lipitor. But now doctors are writing prescriptions for the new drug that is up to ten times more expensive. Just the other day I had an elderly man and his wife come in. He's 85 and she's 79. You should have seen the look on their faces when they saw how much the new prescription was going to cost them. I'd never seen such sticker shock in my life. They're on a fixed income and she nearly broke down in tears.

I asked them to have a seat and wait for a few minutes before leaving. I told them I needed to check on something."

She continued: "Then, I did something I probably shouldn't have done. I called their doctor. Fortunately, I was able to speak with him almost immediately and explained the situation. 'Insurance isn't covering it?' the doctor asked me. And I told him 'No, the new drug is not on the insurance company's formulary, so it is not eligible for coverage.'

"He told me he hadn't realized that when he wrote the prescription for them. He said some studies showed it might be a little more effective so he had decided to give it a try. 'Let's go ahead and just go with the generic Lipitor drug, atorvastatin,' he told me. I said okay, but couldn't hold back from telling him that this couple was not well off, had both been on Lipitor for years, and they could now save a lot of money by using the generic. 'Good point,' he said, and hung up."

Jennifer then asked me, "Doctor Jensen, what do you think should be done in cases like this? Some people can't afford to be switched to the latest and greatest drug, and if they've been on something that has worked well for years, why make the switch just because a new product has ten times the hype at ten times the price backing it up."

It was as though Jennifer had flipped a switch and was ticked off.

"Jennifer," I said, "you asked me if I was frustrated. The truth is, frustrated is too benign a word for how I feel. I am offended at how Big Pharma has been manipulating and gouging the American public for decades. I understand how Big Pharma can influence

the healthcare industry in determining which new medicines are approved and which are shoved aside or even discredited in favor of the new expensive drugs. How is this even possible? It's because Big Pharma has one of the largest, most influential, and most powerful network of lobbyists in Washington, D.C. So, yes, it frustrates me to no end to realize how all this happens. But make no mistake, they are not the only culprits to blame. Doctors play right into their hands with their righteous and pompous view of the world as if they alone can make these decisions. And the insurance companies and pharmacy benefit managers get their hands in the honeypot as well. The whole darn cyclic system drives me crazy!"

"Well, Dr. Jensen, I noticed that the company that manufactures Lipitor quit marketing it because it is no longer a trade name drug protected by a patent. So the new patented medicine does all the advertising and the doctors, for whatever reason, start prescribing it left and right, and the new drug generates huge profits. It's almost like an ATM cash machine. The pharmaceutical manufacturers must be working with insurance companies by working out new discount schedules and incentives for the new drug to be approved and placed on the formulary networks. The doctors seem to naively buy into the patient assistance programs, which initially soften the blow to the cash paying patients. So what really happens is that doctors begin prescribing the new pill that literally costs ten times what the already effective but now generic drug atorvastatin — aka Lipitor — costs. In this manner the newest and most expensive and patent-protected statin gets to replace the former darling of the statin class, and the patient never gets to experience the deeply discounted price of the generic statins. It just doesn't make sense, especially when you think about

people on fixed incomes who struggle constantly to cover their medication costs."

I nodded. "You're absolutely right," I said, "It is confounding and I don't have an answer. But you are certainly raising the right concerns and I applaud you for that. Until we make the public aware of the facts of life in the multibillion-dollar universe of pills, I'm afraid the system Big Pharma has in place will just continue to flourish as it has for the last several decades. Jennifer, I wish I had a better answer for you. But I don't and for what it's worth, I admire you for going to bat for your patients by calling the doctor. You did the right thing."

* * *

That conversation with Jennifer really got me thinking. So I pondered how to really connect the dots. Big Pharma is a monopoly that is filled with both patented and generic drugs. Each year drug companies face numerous patent losses that can affect their bottom-line profit structure.

Pharmaceutical manufacturers rely on their frontline patented products for huge profits. When patents expire, which they do after approximately 15 years, generic versions of those once-patented medications can become available. While consumers benefit from lower prices, losing patent protection can and does expose drug companies to increased competition.

How significant is this? *EvaluatePharma*, an industry trade journal, estimated in 2016 that there could be up to $215 billion in revenue losses due to patent expirations between 2015 and 2020. Take Lipitor, for instance, which lost its exclusivity patent on November 30, 2011, meaning that it was no longer exclusive and could then be distributed by multiple pharmaceutical manufacturers.

When generic manufacturers have access to a drug, they don't incur costs on research and development or advertising. Hence, the price for the same product can drop as much as 95 percent. At that time several companies can compete to sell the drug. Therefore, prices go down and the drug becomes much more affordable to patients.

What Is a Patent?

A patent grants an asset owner the right to exclusive use and distribution of that product for a specified period of time. This exclusivity provides intellectual property protection for that specific amount of time. Once a drug is patented, other companies cannot copy its chemical structure. Legal protection can be extended by applying for peripheral patents that are related to a drug's formulation, production process, method of use, mode of administration, or dosage pattern.

In 1980 the U.S. Supreme Court ruled that biological matter could be patented as part of a formulation. The ruling was made to protect the inventions of biotechnology companies — drugs in this case — from competitors. After all, the development process can be exceedingly expensive, and only a fraction of the drugs that enter the discovery phase get approved and go to market.

How Long Does a Drug Patent Last?

At present a drug patent lasts approximately 15 to 20 years

from the date the pharmaceutical company applies for the patent. In some cases, it can take several years of development and testing before a drug reaches the market.

What Happens When a Drug Patent Expires?

When an exclusive patent expires, other companies are free to create a generic product which will likely command a much lower price. Many patients have asked me about Viagra, an erectile dysfunction drug, or Chantix, a smoking cessation drug. "Hey, Doc, when will the price drop?" They ask because both of these drugs are expensive patented drugs and often erratically covered by insurance plans, if at all. These are good questions and I encourage them.

Rip-off Sales Tactics

I also go out of my way to warn patients about the potential for what I consider "rip-off" drugs. I recall getting very angry when the release of a new fish oil drug started getting prescribed by specialists involved with my patients. This drug can be used to lower triglyceride cholesterol, but for many patients it is little more than a "me-too" drug duplicating inexpensive fish oil products already available to patients as over-the-counter (OTC) supplements. My issue was that this drug was being aggressively marketed to patients on television ads and to doctors in medical journals as something critically important and possibly life-saving. In reality, it was little more than a reformulated fish oil product which could cost patients more than 20 times what the OTC products cost.

My anger was not directed at Big Pharma in this situation — they were simply doing what they've always done. I was furious with my specialist colleagues for not engaging with their patients and providing a full and helpful informed-consent conversation for using a product which had little data demonstrating benefit for patients beyond what OTC fish oils could provide. Doctors must recognize the huge role they can play in helping patients afford the healthcare and medicines they need. Doctors must assume their rightful place as patient advocates and not let Big Pharma gouge the medical marketplace.

A Summary of Expensive Drugs

Here is a rundown of the problem with expensive drugs ruling the day in the world of medication prices:

The notion of the general public is that when an expensive, exclusive drug loses its patent, there should be an opportunity for patients to save some money since generic pharmaceutical companies routinely step in and manufacture a generic drug at a dramatically lower price. But the fact of the matter is that when an expensive patented drug is converted into a generic drug, the pharmaceutical companies have already taken steps to insert into the void created by this conversion a newly patented and "better" expensive drug. When that happens high prices are preserved for the pharmaceutical industry and patients can feel trampled and disregarded. When the billion-dollar blockbuster Lipitor lost its patent and could be produced inexpensively by multiple generic drug manufacturers, patients might have thought that they could finally save some money. But instead Big Pharma reached out its controlling arms and made sure the

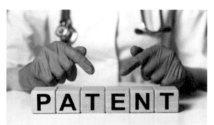

"No man of science wants merely to know. He acquires knowledge to appease his passion for discovery. He does not discover in order to know, he knows in order to discover."

Alfred North Whitehead

billions of dollars used to purchase Lipitor would now be transferred to the next emerging new statin drug. The "statin beast" would continue to be fed by the hidden strategies of the pharmaceutical industry.

With the statin drug family — perhaps more than any other group of drugs — Big Pharma has been able to successfully retain market share in the world of expensive patented drugs. Starting with Mevacor in 1987 and moving on to Pravachol, Zocor, Lipitor, and Crestor, Big Pharma was able to retain huge profits in the statin marketplace despite the availability of much cheaper generic drugs produced along the way. How? Big Pharma paid researchers and cardiologists to do studies which would provide the fodder to elevate the latest and greatest patented statin coming into the market. Cardiologists generally lead the way in cholesterol treatments, and when they abandon a long-used newly converted generic drug, choosing instead to prescribe the latest, newly-patented, and expensive statin (with minimal statistical improvement over the cheaper generic), the rest of the medical community generally follows.

With generic drugs typically of high quality and up to 90 percent cheaper than current patented drugs, I often find myself in the awkward position of discontinuing a colleague's decision to start my patients on the "latest-and-greatest" expensive patented drug simply because my patients cannot afford their cost-sharing responsibility for that particular medication.

Personally, I attempt to prescribe generic drugs as much as possible. Generally they are every bit as effective as their much higher priced counterparts. Unfortunately, there are times when I cannot. I recommend that all patients become knowledgeable about when prescription medications become available as a generic alternative to high-cost medications. Doing so can save a great deal of money with little or no loss in efficacy. In the meantime, I continue to work to find a solution to make effective therapeutic drugs available to everyone who needs them at a price they can afford. Our medication pricing policies contribute mightily to our broken healthcare system.

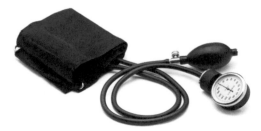

"You never know
how much you really
believe anything until
its truth or falsehood
becomes a matter
of life and death
to you."

–C. S. LEWIS

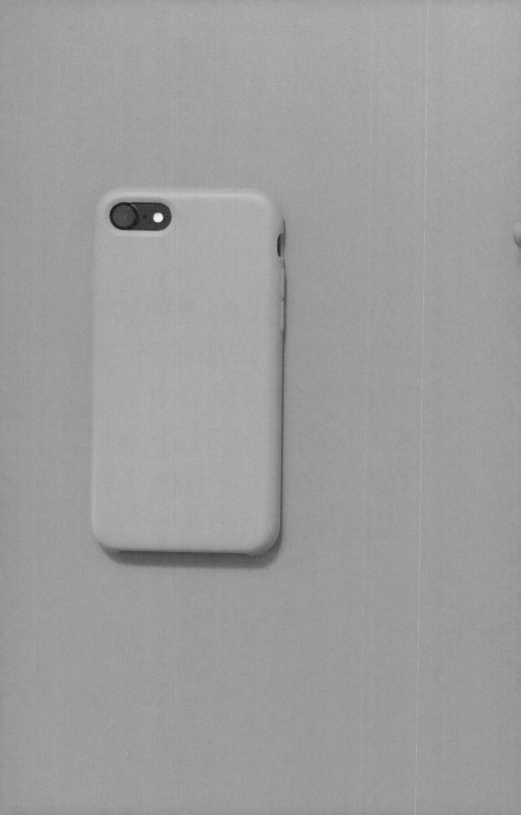

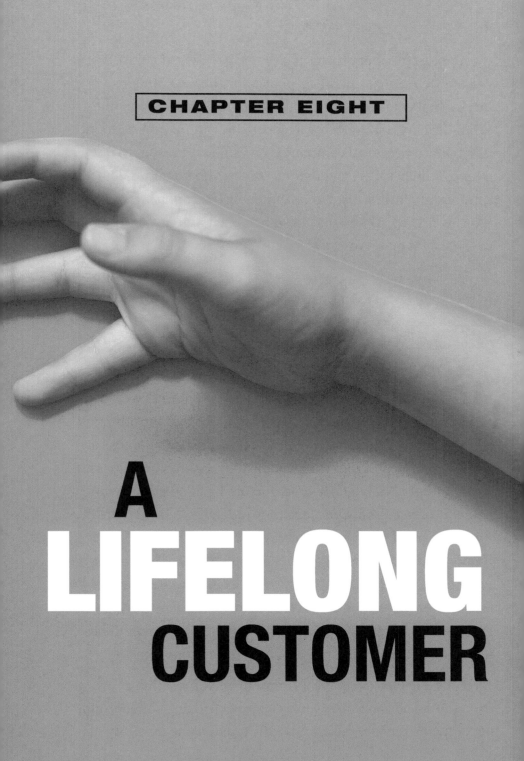

CHAPTER EIGHT

A
LIFELONG
CUSTOMER

A powerful phenomenon has emerged over the past two decades in U.S. healthcare as pharmaceutical companies increasingly market their products directly to the consumer. When I was a young doctor first starting out in medicine, the large pharmaceutical companies had sales representatives who routinely called on doctors, clinics, and hospitals, leaving samples and literature promoting their latest pharmaceutical offerings. They still do that to some extent, but nothing compared to the way it once was.

Directly marketing drugs to the public started in earnest in the 1990s when Viagra came on the scene. Advertising to the consumer quickly became a standard practice for drug companies, and few people could have guessed how huge the impact would be on the practice of medicine.

The idea behind this initiative was that patients would see the ad, and then ask their doctors about that brand-name medication. No longer would pharmaceutical companies rely on physicians to decide if a given product should be discussed with patients. No longer would doctors be allowed to stymie a new product simply because they judged it to be medically unnecessary. If a drug company wanted to increase sales for its hair growth products, a doctor's opinion that such commodities were nothing more than vanity drugs could be circumvented. So direct-to-consumer marketing became the new normal, and the expense of spending millions of dollars daily on national television ads has been passed along to the consumer.

Thus, Big Pharma made its move to take "prescribing" away from the sole discretion of physicians by targeting patients and encouraging them to request specific brand name medications

— whether they were medically needed or not. Drug companies introduced the now-common mantra: "Ask your physician about ..."

So, it's easy to see how direct-to-consumer advertising can increase costs in our healthcare system, but let's discuss how a new twist in this technique is rolling out these days.

* * *

One Patient's Observation

As I entered the exam room Mario looked anxious. "Hey, Doc, do you mind if I ask a question?"

I almost laughed. "Mario, you're here to ask me questions. That's how you get the information you need to be in charge of your health."

Mario continued: "Have you seen the new commercials on television that have the insulin companies encouraging diabetic patients to stick with them for their diabetic needs?"

I looked at Mario and smiled. "Yes, Mario, among other types of meds being advertised on TV, I have noticed that insulin manufacturers have increased their presence, too. Now I'm curious, what television ad are you referring to?"

"Doc, it's the ad by an insulin manufacturer that says if you're using their long-acting insulin, you could also use their short-acting insulin. It seems like the message is that you may be better off sticking with the same company. I was just surprised that they seem to be pushing their diabetic product line as better than that of other companies."

I responded. "Mario, I haven't seen the specific ad you're referring to, but what you probably saw was a pharmaceutical company mimicking marketing strategies used by computer and cell phone corporations. Think about the computer ads for a minute. They also want you to buy their phones and all their accessories. And by the way, purchase your music from them also. They want you to be their fully committed lifelong customer. That strategy is what we are seeing with many medical device companies these days. It would not surprise me to see companies start marketing a full line of needles, lancets, glucose strips, and insulin pumps for diabetics. They're taking a page from another industry."

He interrupted, "Wow!"

"Mario, I think you'll also see that insurance company formularies may be endorsing entire product lines that pharmaceutical companies offer — if the price is right. In fact, with the way insurance companies now operate, it's possible that in the future you may not even have a choice regarding the diabetic line of products you use. That is the cold, hard reality of what is happening in the world of medicine. And it will frustrate patients if the insurance companies switch products on their formularies because of low bids coming from a different pharmaceutical manufacturer."

* * *

Questions to Ponder

What influence should insurance company formularies have on patient and physician choices for medications — or devices for that matter? Who should have a seat at the table when it comes to determining which meds will be included in the most favorable pricing tier of insurance company formularies?

How can insurance companies, pharmaceutical manufacturers, and pharmacy benefit managers (CVS Caremark, Optum Rx, Express Scripts) be held to standards that ensure patient needs are not being ignored?

Is there a risk that patients may end up being nothing more than a pawn on the chess board of medication and device profiteering?

Should formularies be allowed to change mid-year when patients are stuck with their insurance choice through the end of the year?

However you answer these questions, I believe it is a moral imperative that patient needs be kept front and center in the world of essential drugs and medical devices. We are all wise to understand that the pharmaceutical industry has a huge appetite for dollars and control, and monopolizing behaviors are natural outgrowths of such cravings.

In this present-day environment of uncontrolled healthcare costs, strategies must be developed to encourage corporate responsibility that will serve the interests of the common good. With recognition that the dollar-driven policies of Big Pharma have been in place for decades, isn't it time for us to engage in the courageous and difficult conversations which address the necessary balance of ethics and profits?

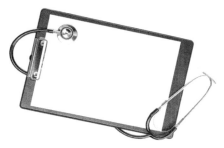

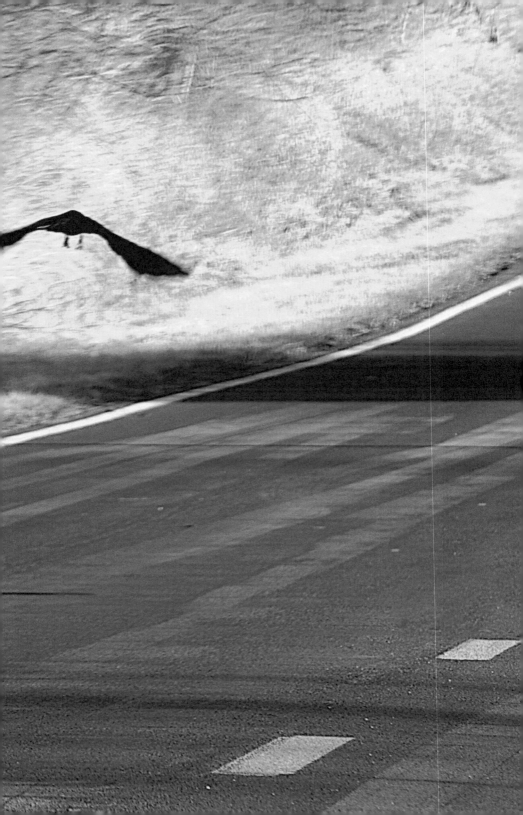

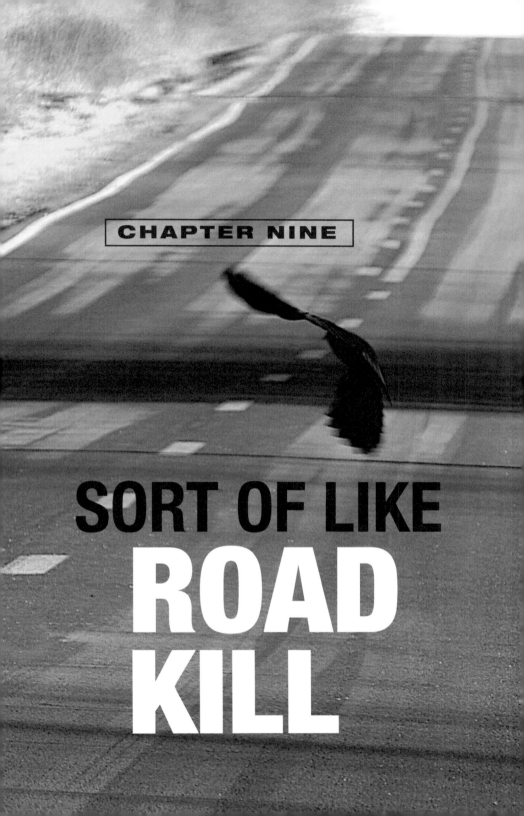

CHAPTER NINE

SORT OF LIKE
ROAD
KILL

We are at a crossroads in our nation in large part because political doublespeak and gridlock continue to disrupt problem-solving efforts, and transparency in policy-making is an almost meaningless term bantered about by politicians. Many patients believe their concerns are of little consequence to politicians and bureaucrats, and that their voices are disregarded.

An impossible labyrinth of billing practices contributes to patient frustration and often leads them to skip life-sustaining investigations and treatments. It is no wonder that a couple of patients confessed to me that they feel "sort of like roadkill" — discarded and ignored. Industry stakeholders, racing toward ever greater healthcare profits, casually snub disenfranchised patients who routinely face the nearly impossible task of navigating an agonizing maze of heartless self-serving agendas designed by insurance conglomerates, management companies, hospital systems, and doctors.

Patients don't feel cared for. They feel abused and lost. Patients don't feel like the center of attention in an industry purportedly created for the welfare of the sick and the hurting. They feel exploited. Too often patients must beg for an explanation for inexplicable bills while yearning for someone to care at least a little about their plight.

How did the business of caring for others come to be so little focused on serving others?

Our healthcare system has a single enormous inborn problem, and it is this: all the major stakeholders — insurance, Big Pharma, software businesses, medical supply and device companies, government agencies, public health departments, hospitals, clinics, doctors, and even patients — generally benefit when the medical-industrial complex is fed more dollars. And the faster the growth, the more profits tend to increase, along with a corresponding decrease in oversight.

The oversimplified argument that a single-payer system will solve our healthcare woes is delusional and will do little to diminish the relentless pursuit of dollars. We can easily observe the lessons that the United Kingdom has learned about the inadequacies of a government-run system of caring for people who suffer real and urgent needs. In fact we don't have to travel any further than our own Veterans Administration system of serving our soldiers to see that a single-payer approach to medical care is no panacea. The essence of optimizing the way we care for the sick and dying is far more complicated than limiting the number of payers to one. It has to do with seeing the "whole" patient, which includes a lot more than just ordering tests, dispensing drugs, or grabbing a scalpel. It has to do with caring about whether patients can actually access the treatment recommended. It has to do with informing patients with understandable words and lessons so that true informed consent can actually be a reality.

The drive for more profits will only be slowed by recognizing the healthcare malfunction for what it is — an ongoing hemorrhage of responsibility on the part of virtually every stakeholder involved. For me personally, forty years of seeing patients has driven home the lesson that "picking off the scab" is sometimes the only way to begin the process of real healing.

Following is a particularly poignant experience I had with a patient who suffered from breast cancer and had limited funds on which to live. My anger exploded on a day when my patient was harmed by a system which had lost its soul.

* * *

I remember well Gladys, who wept in my exam room because she was struggling to choose between paying for her chemotherapy pills or paying the grocery bill. I heard her story and was incensed to learn that her oncologist had switched her cancer pill from a cheap generic to a newly released patented drug — which was structurally similar to the generic, but cost more than twenty times as much. Madder than hell, I marched into my office, closed the door, and called the oncologist.

"What in the world are you doing, Leonard? You told Gladys to stop the tamoxifen, which she could afford and started her on your new-found favorite trade name drug, XYZ? She's in my office crying. I just looked up the two drugs and the XYZ drug you recommended is marginally, if at all, more effective and is classified in the same family of drugs. Leonard, she can't pay her grocery bill, for heaven's sake! Gladys is scared her cancer will kill her if she doesn't do as you told her, but she's also frustrated because she doesn't know how to make ends meet."

Interrupting quickly, Leonard blurted, "Hold on, Scott. Please! I'm sorry. I didn't know finances would be an issue or that her insurance wouldn't cover it. You're right. The new patented drug shows some possible advantages, but nothing dramatic. Please tell her to get back on the tamoxifen. I feel bad. I'm glad you called."

Calming down quickly, I said, "Okay, Leonard. Thanks for taking my call and understanding. Gladys likes you and didn't want to disobey your instructions. I'll tell her. I think you see her next month, and maybe you could reinforce what you just told me."

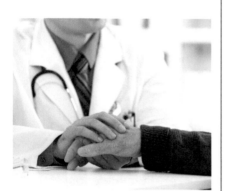

Many patients believe their concerns are of little consequence and that their voices are disregarded.

"Oh, I will certainly do that, Scott. You can count on me." His voice was subdued and apologetic.

After hanging up I was still irritated. "If the new drug isn't a dramatic improvement over the cheap generic tamoxifen," I thought, "why in the world did Leonard even make the switch?" I knew that even though Gladys would breathe a sigh of relief, she would also harbor a doubt as to whether or not she was taking the absolute best drug for her breast cancer. And I was angry because I realized many patients didn't have the relationship Gladys and I shared. Those patients just might choose to skip the groceries and take the new pill.

* * *

The point of this story is not just that doctors contribute mightily to a fractured healthcare system, and that patients must be more than passive bystanders. Unfortunately, a patient needs to be willing to go against his or her physician's advice and insert some desperately needed common sense into a system gone astray. That patient must ask about the specific benefits of a medication and how likely he or she is to be helped by its use.

Patients should investigate a concept known as the NNT — Number Needed to Treat — which can help them determine the likelihood that they will receive a benefit from a particular medicine. Physicians must do a much better job of asking themselves how a specific intervention — a medication, a surgery, or a test — will actually benefit a patient or change a plan of care.

In the end the reason for having doctors, hospitals, insurance companies, and Big Pharma is all about the only legitimate focus of the healthcare industry — THE PATIENT — and we have lost our way. Patients sometimes do feel "sort of like roadkill" — discarded and of little consequence.

TOO MUCH PROFIT

IS BEING MADE AT THE EXPENSE OF UNSUSPECTING PATIENTS.

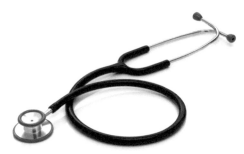

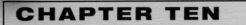

CHAPTER TEN

A LOVE AFFAIR
with
PRE

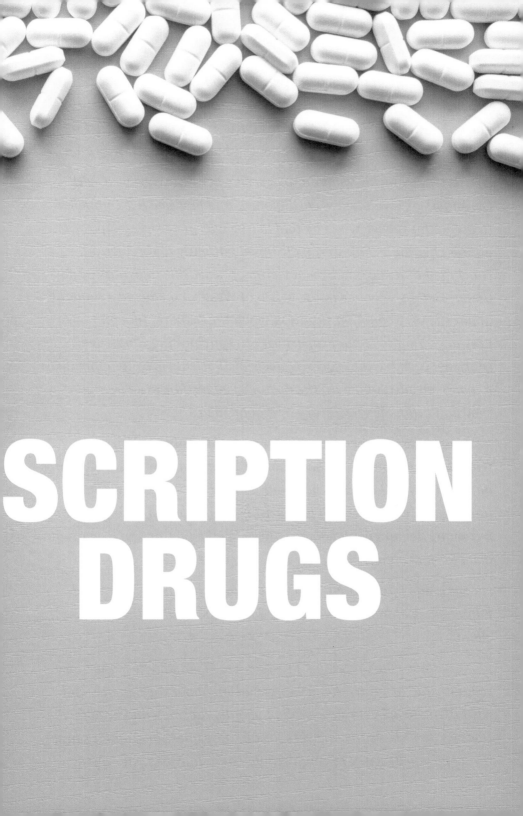

She was one of my favorite patients. So I was taken aback when, before I had even closed the exam room door, Gertrude blurted out her complaint, "Is this Lipitor really necessary? I didn't want to disagree with the heart doctor, but do I have to stay on it?"

Gertrude quickly went on to describe her awkward visit with Dr. Anderson, a renowned cardiologist, and how she felt compelled to accept his advice when he told her he was prescribing Lipitor to address her high cholesterol. I listened patiently and reluctantly concluded that she had been a victim of "scientific bullying" — not an uncommon practice in the world of Western medicine. I thought about the very common situation when the "expert" (doctor) presumes an intellectual superiority to convince the "audience" (patient) to make the "correct" decision. Patients are often inclined to passively go along with the doctor's suggestion, even though they don't think it's necessary or a good idea.

"Gertrude, I'm sorry you had an uncomfortable conversation with Dr. Anderson. He's a good doctor. Doctors often disagree with one another, and we each have our own viewpoint as to what's important. I disagree with his decision to prescribe Lipitor for you, but many doctors would do exactly as he did. Lipitor can be a great drug for lots of folks, but it isn't for everyone."

Gertrude interrupted, "But I'm closing in on ninety years old. I don't want more pills, and I sure don't believe what the TV ads claim."

"Good for you, Gertrude," I responded. "TV and newspapers are certainly full of contradictory information about the benefits and risks of medicines, surgeries, supplements, vaccines, and even foods. Doctors don't have the answers for all these questions, and it's best if you, as much as you're comfortable, take charge of your own

health. So please don't be offended by Dr. Anderson's prescription
for Lipitor. He's just used to pulling out his prescription pad if the
cholesterol number is higher than he likes. I must confess, Gertrude,
lots of doctors seem to have a love affair with prescription drugs.
But you should never hesitate to check with your pharmacist about
your prescriptions. They're the real experts on taking pills. But
to get back to your question — no, you don't have to stay on the
Lipitor. I sure wouldn't."

* * *

Common sense in 21st century healthcare will have to come
from the combined efforts of patients and doctors. As much as
physicians are inclined to view their own perspective as the
superior one, this is often not the case. Physician arrogance is
part of the reason our healthcare system is broken and why
patients often feel like pawns on a chess board. The frequency
with which patients feel pushed by doctors to take medicines
is growing rapidly. The casual manner with which doctors
prescribe drugs is especially concerning because appropriate
"informed consent" seldom occurs. Few patients are told that
statin drugs used to lower cholesterol can actually increase the
risk of developing diabetes in some patients.

I remember having to call a neurologist, Dr. Julie Risky, about
a mutual patient with mild dementia. She was absolutely certain
Archie needed to be on donepezil, a drug used for dementia
patients. This drug has had mixed reviews from physicians,
patients, and families, and I seldom recommend it. When Dr. Risky
got on the phone, I suggested stopping the donepezil that she had
prescribed for Archie. Before I could explain my reasoning, she
forcefully launched into a speech about how she was the specialist

and what business did I have telling her what to do. When she finally took a breath, I quickly said, "Archie is pooping in his pants and this never happened until you started the donepezil. His family is now thinking he may have to be moved into a nursing home because his wife can't manage this new problem. I just thought that it would be a good idea to stop the donepezil and see if the stool incontinence issue might go away."

Dr. Risky's tone changed abruptly and she said, "Oh, I see," and told me she would call the family and stop the donepezil. A month later I saw Archie and his wife, the incontinence had stopped, and so had the discussions about moving Archie to a nursing home.

Doctors often display a special affinity for pills, and prescribing them gives tangible purpose to their efforts. Patients must beware that this is a big part of the overall problem of our fractured healthcare system. Patients contribute much needed common sense to the highly complex process of medication management. Doctors should remember that.

Together patient and physician need to weigh the benefits and the risks of any proposed prescription drug, and share the responsibility of deciding what makes the most sense. Patients confront a difficult task in declining the well-intentioned recommendation of a healthcare provider, but they must learn to respect their own assessment and weigh in on the plan of care as it is being developed.

The over-prescribing of drugs by doctors has been described in multiple medical journals as the most common unnecessary intervention in the U.S., and this has been going on for decades. Despite containing less than five percent of the world's population, the U.S. consumes far more prescription drugs than any other nation. Numerous studies have concluded that the danger associated with prescription drugs increases dramatically with the number of pills used.

A related but separate issue focuses on the needs of patients who suffer from multiple medical problems and require a daily regimen of dozens of pills. These individuals benefit immensely from having a committed team advocating for them. They need family members, local pharmacists, and home nursing services to work together to coordinate and optimize their health. It is important to note that such a team approach will actually reduce healthcare costs in the long run. But here again, much of the common sense that makes for high quality healthcare will come from patients and families.

While doctors certainly have the expertise and training on the science of medications and the physiology of the body, patients need to champion their own health and never relinquish this responsibility. At the end of the day, they are the ones who must endure the fruits of medical interventions, good or bad. Doctors do not.

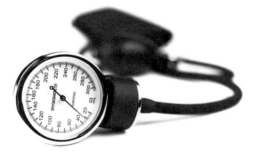

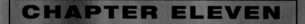

CHAPTER ELEVEN

PULLING BACK the CURTAIN

"Doc, I'm mad as hell!"

I noticed Fred was holding a hospital bill in his hand and I suspected what was coming. Unfortunately, I had seen this many times — the unexpected sticker shock of a procedure or a hospital bill that blindsided a patient.

"What's up, Fred?"

"My wife had a kidney stone. We went to the emergency room. Barb was throwing up, crying, and gasping with pain. After a couple of hours in the ER, the nurses took her to a hospital room, where we stayed most of the day. She was still in a lot of pain, but slowly it got better. Finally, after 18 hours in the hospital, the doctor said we could go home. Over the next few days Barb was back on her feet and feeling normal. We never did see any stone in her urine. Then a few weeks later we get this massive hospital bill. What the hell for!"

He handed me the bill. I didn't say anything, but scanned it, and I wasn't surprised. It was as I had guessed.

"Dammit, Doc! We have complete coverage, a full-on Cadillac plan that is supposed to take care of everything. If we're hospitalized, it's supposed to cover the entire thing. What the hell is this?" Fred's anger was boiling over.

So I asked, "Fred, did anybody actually tell you that Barbara was being admitted into the hospital?"

He thought for a moment. "Well … no. I guess not specifically. We started in the emergency room, where they told us she had a kidney stone. The nurses made it clear that controlling the pain might help the stone pass on its own. And then they moved Barb up to the second floor to a newer part of the hospital."

"By chance, did they mention anything about 'observation'?"
I asked.

"Well, yeah, now that you mention it I think I remember them
saying they needed to observe her to make sure she did okay. That
sure made sense to us. Barb was truly miserable. I think the nurse
said something about transitioning us from the ER to a room to
keep a close eye on her. I think that's what they said ... but honestly,
Doc, they were using a lot of words I'm not used to."

"Fred, I hate to be the one to break this to you — but this bill
you received indicates that they did not actually admit Barb into
the hospital."

"Well, they sure as heck did. I didn't spend the day at the beach!
First, it was the ER, and then it was upstairs to a room with her
own toilet. And there was a boatload of paperwork to fill out and
sign. Doc, I was there the whole time with her. There were signs all
over that said hospital this and hospital that, so don't tell me Barb
wasn't in the hospital!"

"I see. Fred, it looks like the hospital staff did not actually
formally admit Barb, but rather, they assigned her to observation
status."

"Which means what?" he asked.

"It means Barbara was not actually formally admitted into
the hospital. And that means she was billed under a different code.
Your insurance coverage would likely be more favorable if she had
indeed been admitted into the hospital. But observational status
sometimes means that patients will have to pay more of the bill out
of their own pocket."

Fred's face flushed! "Doc, that's bullshit! You know it and I know it — they're just playing games."

"I do know that," I answered, and I knew my voice was laden with resignation.

"So, why the bait and switch?" asked Fred.

"Just like everyone else, hospitals have to pay their bills, and some of the hospitals' payers are allowed to pay such deeply discounted rates that hospitals look for alternative ways to classify or code the cares they provide. Obamacare and government programs have made things more difficult for a lot of hospitals. So, to offset low reimbursement rates, hospital administrators look for a different way to charge for short-term care — for example, patients with kidney stones. Financial and coding wizards came up with 'observational care' protocols, which can often increase hospital revenues.

Fred was starting to get it, but he clearly was still frustrated, so I continued. "Insurance plans vary tremendously. Sometimes using 'observational care' status instead of an 'admission' is an advantage for hospitals but not for patients. Sometimes it might not affect the patient but will still be better for the hospital. Fred, hospitals have entire departments devoted to optimal coding and charging and collecting."

"How am I supposed to know any of that?" he objected.

"They're supposed to inform you," I said, and then added, "fully and understandably inform you."

"Well, they didn't. Or if they did, I certainly didn't understand it. I just wanted them to do whatever they needed to do to help Barb. So now I get stuck with a damn bill for a couple thousand dollars because of a technicality? Doc, I got scammed!"

I didn't know what to tell him. He and Barbara had experienced, full-on, what our broken healthcare system has become.

"Fred, I'd recommend you dispute it. Explain the situation, what you were told and what wasn't made clear, and let the hospital billing folks know what you thought was going on. Who knows, maybe someone will work with you on this. Try to negotiate it down."

"But we had full coverage — I shouldn't have to pay a thing!"

"I know, I get it."

* * *

Questions to Consider

How can we pull back the curtain regarding medical charges so that total transparency becomes a reality, and patients don't feel they are being scammed and have to constantly play defense?

Let's face it, being hospitalized for most people is a little like buying a car. You don't do it often enough to become really good at it. How are patients to know that what they think is happening — i.e., a hospital admission — is not really happening, but instead a transfer from the emergency room to 'observational care' is taking place because that move will garner greater revenue for the hospital?

Billing transparency is absolutely necessary and the lack of it has been a huge healthcare problem for the last several decades. Elective procedures can be planned, but emergency situations cannot. People aren't interested in negotiating or asking questions if they or a loved one is having a heart attack. Insurance companies could also be far more transparent, but generally they are hyper-focused on marketing and selling policies. Worrying about whether or not a patient fully understands an insurance contract is of less concern for many insurance agents than making sure they are hitting their quotas.

How do we motivate insurance companies, hospital systems, clinics, and doctors to be truly transparent and fix the problem Fred and Barbara experienced?

Can our fractured healthcare industry be fixed without calling out "the man behind the curtain"?

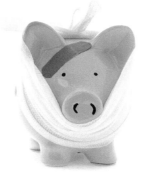

"FINANCIAL RUIN FROM MEDICAL BILLS IS ALMOST EXCLUSIVELY AN AMERICAN DISEASE."

—Roul Turley

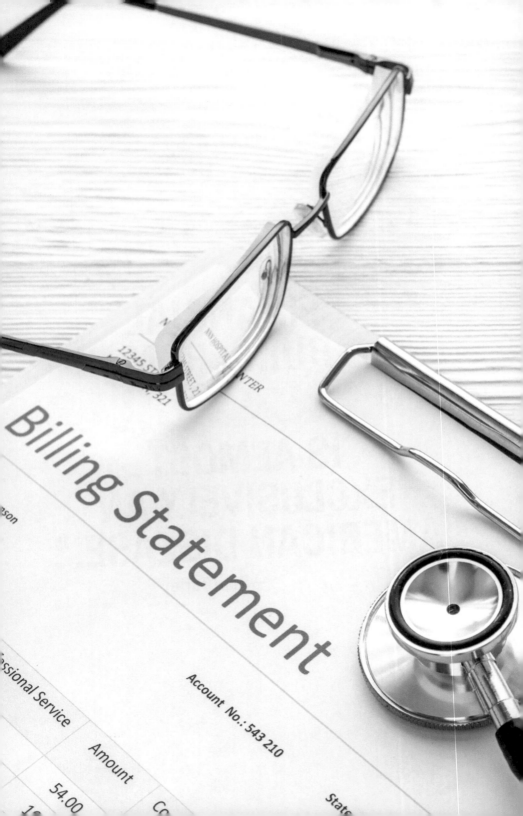

CHAPTER TWELVE

BECAUSE
THEY
CAN

2/01/2021

5432

14

One of the most difficult issues facing hard-working men and women today, especially those with families, is the fact that they have no frame of reference for what standard medical procedures should cost. This is particularly true for those who have no medical insurance, or have an insurance plan with a very high deductible. As a result, patients frequently will not seek medical attention when they really should. Unfortunately, this delay often allows a straightforward problem to become life-threatening and hugely expensive, because, quite simply, the medical intervention came too late. Exorbitant bills have many unintended and unfortunate consequences.

* * *

The voice on the other end of the phone was shaky. I could tell something was wrong and I wondered why Andrea sounded so distressed. This was not the happy, positive young soccer mom I usually see at my clinic.

"Hi Andrea, what's up?"

I sensed her hesitation before she said, "Dr. Jensen, I know it isn't fair to take up your time for this, but I didn't know anyone else who I trust enough to ask. The truth is, I just don't know what to do."

"I'll be happy to help in any way I can."

"Dr. Jensen, it's about something that happened last weekend. Our son Timmy cut himself, and Jim and I thought it looked bad. Since it happened on Sunday, we weren't sure where to go, so we took Timmy to the hospital. Fortunately, the doctor said it wasn't too bad of a cut, and he closed it up with some kind of 'super-glue.' Then he sent us on our way. He only spent a couple of minutes with

us, but when we got the bill today for $2,000, I just broke down and cried. My husband, Jim, called the hospital to see if there was some kind of mistake, but the billing person said it was correct and we had thirty days to pay. Seriously, Doctor Jensen, the ER doctor could not have been in the room more than five minutes. How can this be?"

I answered, "Andrea, I wish I had something else to tell you, but all I can say is they sent you that bill because they can. I know that's not a good answer, but it's the truth and that's just the way it is. I'm sorry. I wish our clinic had been open, because we could have avoided this. Typically, hospital-based care is five to ten times more expensive than clinic care. Andrea, in the future you might even want to use a "quick clinic" to sort of triage the situation. I am so sorry this happened. I think you should call the hospital billing department and see if they will work with you on this. Those folks are usually kind, understanding, and want to help get issues resolved."

* * *

Unfortunately, stories like Andrea's play out thousands of times each and every day throughout America, and I believe it is because the Relative Value System used in medical billing is flawed. Its comparative standards and guidelines try to match time allotment and required expertise necessary for medical procedures with pricing formulas. It is far from a perfect system and needs to be addressed.

But there are other immediate problems in the world of healthcare coding and billing. A mentor of mine once told me that if I was unsure a patient had sprained or fractured a wrist, it would be best to diagnose a fracture. The mentor went on to say that three good things happen with such an approach: 1) physician reimbursement is higher, 2) malpractice risk is lower, and 3) patients are happier, because if a fracture is not actually present, the patient will get better more quickly than expected and few patients complain about that. Virtually every specialty has similar coding problems which can arise when patients are assigned exaggerated and higher paying diagnostic codes.

Similar situations arise with the diagnosis of borderline diabetes, very mild asthma, or early kidney disease. There is no question that some physicians like to code these diagnoses in the chart, even though it may be detrimental to patients (more patient hassles with future insurance applications, DOT exams, flight physicals, etc.). These diagnoses can be like the "goose that lays the golden egg" for a doctor, because patients can be seen more frequently with briefer visits and keep a doctor's appointment schedule filled. Additionally, the physician may be credited with high-quality care simply because the established disease is considered "well-controlled" — when in reality the disease is simply in a very early stage.

Questions to Ponder

How can medical charges be integrated into a more normal market-based standard using comparative models with other professions?

How can patients avoid the shock and dismay of large bills that have no rational explanation?

How can patients be allowed to "shop" for better prices in the world of healthcare? (We can often shop for elective procedures, but emergencies call for action, not a discussion of prices.)

How can oversight be implemented so that the use of exaggerated diagnostic codes is avoided? (Some clinics stopped using diagnosis and procedural codes completely and simply use credit card payments on a flat rate per fifteen minute blocks of time. This works for some medical issues, but falls far short of being a perfect solution.)

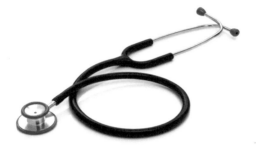

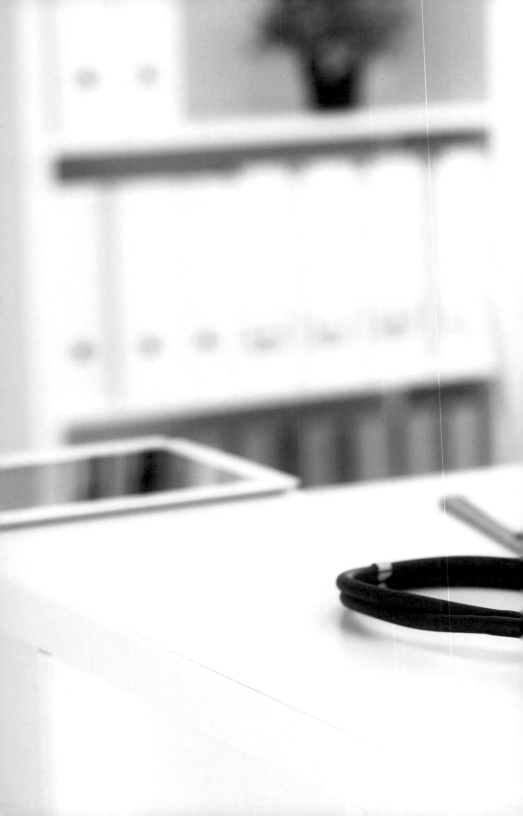

CHAPTER THIRTEEN

WHEN DOCTORS GET IT WRONG

Logan was a delightful, unpretentious, 13-year-old on the cusp of puberty. We had just had a nice visit discussing her classes at school. I reassured her that her ankle was only sprained and not broken. She would get better quickly if she laid off soccer for the next ten days. I always enjoyed seeing Logan because she was disarmingly candid and seemed not even to realize it. She was her own person and didn't try to be someone she wasn't. She didn't deflect questions, but answered them simply and succinctly in her own wonderful way. I remember thinking that her candor and honesty were precious and that I hoped she would never lose those qualities.

I looked at her dad and said, "Bill, you must be very proud of your daughter."

He smiled and said, "You bet I am, Doc."

Pleased, but slightly embarrassed, Logan blurted, "I need to use the bathroom. Is that okay?"

Bill and I both nodded and out the door she went.

And there we sat. Bill's gaze trailed after her. The room was quiet.

"Everything all right, Bill?" I asked.

He smiled and took a deep breath. "Yeah. I think your comment sort of caught me off guard."

"How so?" I asked.

Struggling with how best to respond, Bill stammered, "I don't know, Doc. I guess it's been a long time since I thought about being 'proud' of her. I mean, yes, she's a great kid and she's doing well. But I've spent years just hoping she might somehow have some semblance of a normal life. It's a little stunning to hear you talk about her as if there's no problem."

"I'm not sure I understand, Bill," I responded. "What do you mean about hoping Logan might have a 'semblance of a normal life' and 'as if there's no problem'?"

"Doc, you do know she's been diagnosed as autistic, don't you?"

I stared at Bill in stunned silence.

"Who made that diagnosis?" I blurted. "Surely no one here in this clinic!"

It was Bill's turn to be a little surprised, "I thought you were just being kind," he commented. "You mean you didn't know what the specialist said several years ago? You've really been thinking she's normal?"

"Bill, when it comes to human personalities, I don't know what 'normal' is, but if you're asking if I think your daughter is healthy, smart, and doing just fine, I say, absolutely. She's a delight and has a refreshingly direct approach in the way she communicates. She says what she thinks and makes no apologies for her bluntness. What's wrong with that?"

"You don't think she's a little odd?" he asked sheepishly.

"No, I don't," I said matter-of-factly.

"Really?" Bill was not the emotional type, but I could hear his voice cracking. It was as if everything inside him wanted that to be true, but he couldn't quite buy into my viewpoint.

"Doc, we were told awhile back that Logan showed signs of autism and was somewhere on the 'spectrum.' When the psychiatrist said those words, Logan's mother and I were devastated. We trained ourselves to expect the worst and never get too thrilled by her achievements or dreams. We promised ourselves we would do everything we could to shelter her from awkward or

embarrassing situations. That's what the counselors told us would be best for Logan. We always waited in fear for the other shoe to drop. I think we did a good job with her, but..."

"But what?" I asked. "She's her own self. She hears the beat of a different drummer at times! So what? I like the way she lives her life without being locked into the same old trap of insecurity many of us battle every day."

He thought about it for a moment. "She certainly sees the world in her own 'Logan' sort of way. She's a loner, but thankfully when she's around others, she does okay. She's no extrovert, but I think she's pretty functional."

"That's bullshit, Bill. Logan is a wonderful young lady and you and your wife are doing a good job raising her. You don't need to be wondering about functionality with her."

I continued: "Let me say this straight, Bill. I don't believe for a minute that Logan is autistic or anywhere close to it. She may have some idiosyncrasies, but who doesn't? I think we call that being 'original.' But rest assured, Logan is wonderfully made and one-of-a-kind. Celebrate that."

Those words hit home, and Bill blinked away some tears while studying his shoes.

"Doc, we never told anyone about the diagnosis. I didn't want to believe it, but what do I know? I'm no expert when it comes to kids. We sure didn't want to drug her up like they recommended, so we just struggled along trying to do the best we could. That's partly why we started coming here — to give Logan a fresh start without the label following her everywhere. Once the specialty clinic tagged her as autistic, that pretty much colored everything that happened there. They made us feel anxious, and the endless *questionnaires we had to fill out drove us a little crazy."*

"Bill, I don't know what the situation was when autism was raised as a diagnostic consideration, and it's obviously a huge deal for many children and their families. But having been Logan's doctor for several years now, and seeing her with the strep throats, sprained ankles, and the occasional cough gives me some basis for an opinion. And I've gotta tell you I've never observed anything that would make me put her 'on the spectrum' of autism."

The room was still and I knew there was a confession that needed to be made.

"Bill, doctors are not infallible. Like everyone else, in the pressure and flow of the demands we can get things wrong. Premature conclusions can cause us to misinterpret the data. Sometimes what we see as signs and symptoms of a problem are just completely wrong. We make misdiagnoses. Sadly, with autism on the rise, a label like that can too readily be assumed to be the truth, when in reality, it was simply a physician's misinterpretation of the signs, symptoms, and circumstances. And when we get it wrong, a misdiagnosis can become a lifelong imprisonment that denies hopes and dreams, and too often gives rise to a horrifying self-fulfilling prophecy."

"Doc, I feel terrible. My wife and I have lived under the shadow of this since Logan started school. The needless anxiety and misguided worry ... "

Bill couldn't go on. His shoulders shook. "What have we done to her?" He choked out the words.

I looked at him and said, "Bill, don't put that on yourself. I understand the frustration, anger even — it makes me mad for you — but if it has caused you to be more considerate and more attentive to her needs, then regardless of how misguided that diagnosis was, you have funneled it into powerful care and love for your daughter. I don't see any damage in that."

"Yeah, but still — what did we do to her by living in fear about her future and never daring to dream of who she might become?"

"You've loved your kid, Bill, and you've done the best for her with the information you had at hand. Leave it at that and move forward. Look, living with the notion that your daughter's uniqueness was autism is on my profession, not you. We've got our biases and sometimes that translates into tragic misdiagnoses. We do our best, most of the time. And somedays, our best just isn't good enough. When we get it wrong, our blunders can ruin lives. But Bill, that hasn't happened with Logan, and I am incredibly grateful for that."

Just then, Logan came bounding back in and plopped right back up on the end of the exam table.

"Well, it's lucky for you, Logan, that it's only a sprain, nothing broken and no permanent damage," I reminded her with a smile.

"It doesn't hurt that bad, Doctor. I'll be fine."

"I know you will!" I said and smiled in agreement.

Bill was beaming, looking very much relieved. "Thanks, Doc, that's good news! I'm not sure who got the most out of this visit, Logan or me, but I'm sure glad we came in."

He gave his little girl a big hug, and out the door they went.

* * *

Not all stories of misdiagnosis end as well as Logan's. Inaccurate data leads to wrong diagnoses. Skewed algorithms, rigid administrative policies, and hypersensitivity to certain symptoms or trends can all contribute to misdiagnosis, especially in a pediatric patient.

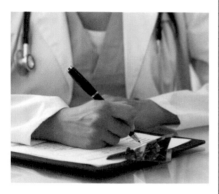

"Everybody is a genius. But if you judge a fish by its ability to climb a tree it will live its whole life believing that it is stupid."
—Albert Einstein

What happens when a physician makes a misdiagnosis? How does it affect a patient, a family, or even a community? That's hard to say, because each given situation is different. But when a doctor has an unrecognized bias that comes into play in caring for a patient, that bias can powerfully dismantle the dreams and hopes of a lifetime. And if such prejudices are borne of political pressures or bureaucratic egos, our healthcare system suffers mightily — and its brokenness is amplified.

However, one aspect of our imperfect method of caring for the sick and healing the hurting is clear: the starting point must be the well-being and empowerment of the patient. We cannot allow Big Pharma or Big Government to have too large a role in how a patient is served.

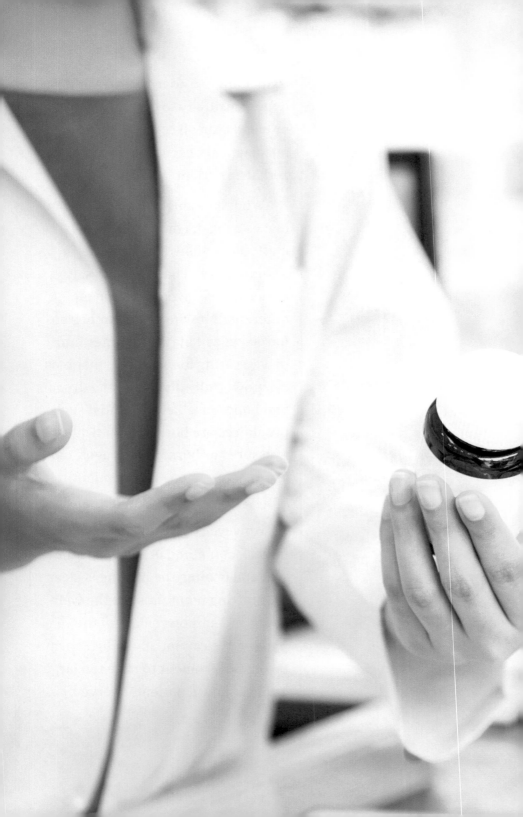

CHAPTER FOURTEEN

PHARMACISTS MATTER

"Paul," I said, as I entered the room and reached out to shake his hand, "you're doing everything right. Your lab tests are remarkable, and I am especially impressed with your cholesterol. I don't have any new suggestions other than to keep on doing what you're doing."

Paul was beaming. "Doc, thanks for the good news, but I do want to ask you a question. Suzanne, my pharmacist, said I should talk to you about maybe trying a different blood pressure medicine. She wrote it down and here's her note. She said that you might be all for it because it has less 'bedroom' side effects on men — if you know what I mean."

I looked at the note and nodded. "I think Suzanne is absolutely right. Her suggestion could definitely reduce the likelihood for erectile dysfunction, and I appreciate the fact that the two of you have the kind of relationship that works together to solve problems. Well done, Paul, and please thank Suzanne when you see her next."

"I sure will," he said, and was on his way to get his prescription filled.

* * *

There is an important takeaway lesson from Paul's story, and that is the value of *relationship*. Paul's pharmacist, Suzanne, took a personal interest in the best possible successful outcome for him. I have seen this dynamic in effect hundreds of times over the years, and I believe that it is a critical component of effective patient care.

My frustration is with the big insurance companies pushing patients to abandon their local pharmacists in favor of mail-

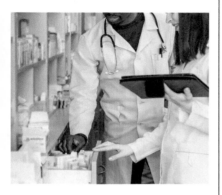

Teaming up with a pharmacist benefits patients in a big way. Relationship matters!

order or big-box pharmacies which are volume driven and much less patient focused. Big insurance companies team up with Big Pharma to drive patients away from their local pharmacy. This is problematic on multiple fronts.

Local pharmacies do a terrific job making certain that patients understand correct dosages and when to take medications. It is not unusual for them to identify errors made by prescribing physicians. Their help and instructions are invaluable and play an integral role in achieving the best possible outcome for patients.

Teaming up with a pharmacist benefits patients in a big way. **Relationship matters!**

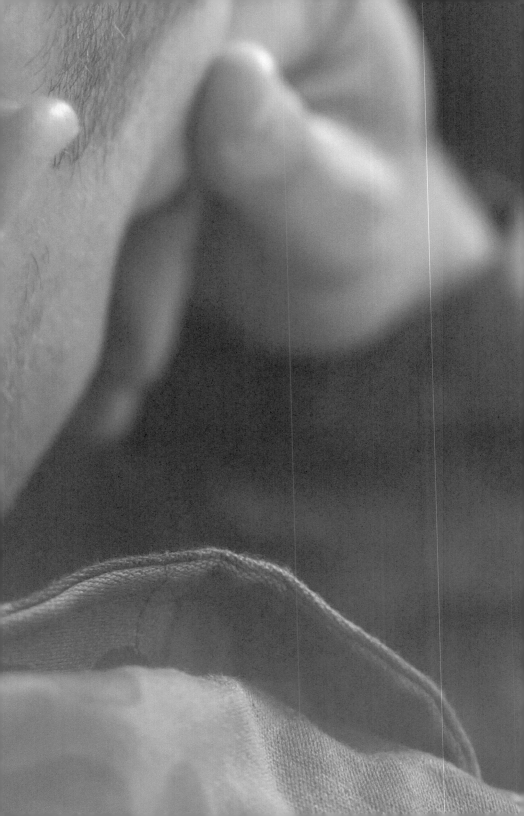

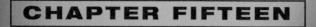

CHAPTER FIFTEEN

A SOLDIER'S TOUGHEST BATTLE

I remember feeling a horrid sense of "you've got to be kidding me" when he unexpectedly disclosed that he had struggled with post-traumatic stress disorder — PTSD — for forty years, and had recently attempted suicide. He told me about his mental demons, and that after his mother died he had moved north to settle his affairs and prepare to once and for all end his private, painful war.

I wondered how I had not picked up on his inner conflict in our long-ago visits. Why had I not recognized the powerful pain that Pete was facing all alone? I had taken care of him for twenty-five years, but I had never seen his torment.

I asked him, "Do you want to tell me about it?"

"Yeah, Doc, I think I'd like to."

And he did. His story was astonishing, not because of gruesome battlefield details, but for the grisly mental trauma and pain he had borne. Here is what he told me:

> *Doc, I had been in Vietnam for about a year, and my responsibilities focused on the prisoner apprehension program. I traveled across the country delivering or picking up prisoners, getting them where they needed to be for various legal proceedings.*
>
> *I never saw it coming. The mission was supposed to be routine, with three of us going to pick up two prisoners, both U.S. soldiers, and transporting them back to base camp. We found out along the way that one of the prisoners was accused of killing another soldier in his platoon — which was weird — and the whole situation turned out to be anything but mundane.*
>
> *So we picked up these two guys and were flying back*

to base on board a Huey helicopter when we were shot down very close to the Cambodian border. The pilot did a great job of landing the burning Huey, and none of us was seriously injured, so we were able to hit the ground running to get away from the flames as fast as possible. But everything changed when the helicopter exploded. The nearby trees caught fire and roared. We could just as well have put out a news bulletin that we were in the area, and sure enough, North Vietnamese soldiers realized an opportunity and rushed to grab it.

I figured hostiles would be spreading out, trying to outflank us, and things would heat up quickly. I wasn't wrong. Soon enough we could hear soldiers scurrying about the jungle, moving toward us, and though I didn't speak North Vietnamese, I knew these weren't friends coming to help.

I got so nervous, Doc, to think I was maybe just a few minutes away from being dead, or maybe even worse, about to become a POW in a North Vietnamese prison camp. I was actually too scared to think. I simply reacted and moved away from the voices and toward where I thought we might find a South Vietnamese base camp. Me and my guys moved as quietly and quickly as we could. I was so filled with fear I thought I'd throw up. I felt even worse when I saw how my buddies were acting. They were taking the situation in stride and doing what needed to be done. But there I was, scared silly.

Doctor Jensen, I kid you not. There in the middle of the Vietnam jungles, I was in danger, on foot, outnumbered, but most of all disgusted with myself for not being brave.

The next three days were pure hell, and we did our best to avoid the enemy. Based on voices, sounds, and locations, we thought they probably outnumbered us by about ten to one. We couldn't give our prisoners guns, so they wouldn't be much help. We were in a real pickle.

We desperately tried to connect with friendlies — South Vietnamese or American soldiers — but we didn't know where best to look. We could tell the enemy was tracking us and slowly closing in. Time wasn't on our side. We were in territory we had never seen before and couldn't know what was on the other side of the next hill. We did everything we could to mask our movements and positions, but at night when things got quiet, we could sometimes hear North Vietnamese soldiers talking and barking orders. They weren't far away.

It was the third night out when things got really hairy. It was pitch black — no moon, no stars — and I was doing the final two-hour watch before dawn. I could hear North Vietnamese soldiers nearby, and it sounded like they were advancing. We had taken cover on high ground under a rock outcropping and been hunkered down for about six hours. We lit no fires, and conversation was nothing more than a few whispered observations and instructions. I worried my breathing was too noisy. My guts were jelly. I prayed for a miracle. I thought the end was near.

I wish I could forget that night, Doc, but I can't. My throat was so dry I couldn't swallow. I wanted to cry like a baby. My finger never left the trigger of the machine gun I cradled — not for two whole hours. There was a jungle to my left and a swamp behind me. I could hear North Vietnamese soldiers coming. Their voices carried in the night. I didn't know what they were saying. I hated myself for thinking it, but I thought about calling out and surrendering. I wanted to live — I didn't want to die in a gun battle I knew we couldn't win.

And just when surrender seemed like the best option, I melted with fear at the thought of being a POW. And then I decided that I would fight and die rather than live as a prisoner. All night long I flip-flopped between giving up and dying. I knew I was a coward, and I hated knowing. I was so damn scared!

The night went on forever, but finally sunlight cracked the eastern sky, and my buddies and I roused our prisoners and started moving to the east toward what we thought was friendly territory.

That morning I was point man, which meant that I did recon in front of the others. I saw movement about a hundred yards in front of me, and I jerked my rifle to my shoulder, sighting where the movement had been. I saw a soldier with a South Vietnamese insignia on his right shoulder, so I hollered at the top of my lungs, "Choo hoy," which meant "my friend." The soldier turned and saw me and yelled likewise. We approached each other, and when he clapped me on the shoulder, I fell to my knees and shook.

Everything bubbled out and I could barely speak. I mumbled. My eyes watered. My South Vietnamese protector seemed to understand. He said nothing, just sort of stood by keeping me safe. My buddies arrived at my position with the two prisoners in hand, and eight more South Vietnamese soldiers joined us. Everybody seemed way more in control than me, and that made me feel even worse. I remember thinking that I had never realized what a coward I was.

We all marched out of the jungle together, and it seemed that with each step I regained some composure. We arrived safely at a base camp in a few hours.

Doc, I never ever talked about my fear with anyone. I was ashamed. I finished my tour of duty and got the hell out of the military.

After a long moment I said, "Pete, that's an amazing story. I am blown away."

"Doc," he replied, "when I left Vietnam I thought all the bad stuff was over and I would just get on with living my life. I was so wrong. Little did I know my toughest struggles were yet to come. Soon after getting back home, I started experiencing odd thoughts — guilt trips, I guess — and they wouldn't leave me alone. My mind was like a battlefield, and something was always chasing me. I couldn't get away, and whenever I tried to hide by thinking of something other than Vietnam, these toxic accusations found me and taunted me.

"Over time I realized the source of my torment was my gutlessness during that mission in Nam, and there was nothing I could do about it. I couldn't get away from the guilt. I was a mess and kept getting worse; I had a demon in my head, and I couldn't do anything about it. I hated myself. And yet there was Mom, needing me, living with me. I had to be there for her, stay alive for her. But once she was gone, there really was nothing stopping me *from ending it all by just blowing out my brains."*

"Pete, I had no idea," I answered.

"How could you? I kept those thoughts locked tight in my head. Forty years after I almost died in Vietnam, my Mom's death opened a door I had worked very hard at keeping shut. Her passing gave me a weird kind of permission to go where I was afraid to go, didn't want to go, but felt I had to go. I knew I couldn't stay where I was — my demons were winning. Something snapped. Did you notice you never saw me again after Mom died? I wanted to talk with you about my screwed-up thinking because I knew I was in trouble. But I couldn't do it."

Laying my hand on his shoulder, I whispered, "Pete, I wish I had been there for you. I thought you had simply retired to your cabin up north."

"You couldn't have known," he said. "I was already pretty far down the road — miserable and confused and scared, pretty much holding everything in until Mom left to meet her Maker."

"Pete, you were so good to your mom, always making sure her every need was taken care of. She may not have told you, but she told me many times how proud she was of you."

"Thanks. You know, Doc, I remember when she asked you to throw her in the river because she was too old to be of any use. I still chuckle about that every once in a while."

"She was a little stubborn, but her heart was always in the right place," I said.

"Anyway, in those days, if I wasn't taking care of Mom, all I could think about was enemy soldiers wanting to kill me in the

pitch black of night and me being a coward while my buddies were brave. Then Mom passed and the thoughts got worse and worse until they just took over. Looking back, I had already started to die. I just needed to pull the trigger, but when it got down to doing it, I couldn't."

"I'm sure glad you didn't, Pete," I said.

"Thank God I called the vets hospital. Those folks saved my life. I spent a lot of time there. They told me I had a sort of nervous breakdown. A psychiatrist explained why I was feeling what I was feeling, and the counselors helped me look at bravery and courage in a different light. I was pretty mixed up, and it was really important for me to learn that fear isn't the same as being a coward. And sure enough, I slowly got better. I let go of a lot of poison inside my head and quit feeling so guilty, and now that I'm back, I'm here to stay."

We sat there in silence for a few moments, and then I offered, "Pete, I'm sure glad some good people were there to help you."

When Pete's mom died, I assumed he had done what he had dreamed of doing, moving to the north woods and enjoying a slower pace — more hunting and fishing during the day, more campfires and stars in the night. But that's not what he did. He didn't go up north and enjoy the smell of pine trees and the beckoning of loons. No, Pete retired to his cabin to withdraw from an unwinnable contest with his private demons.

Thankfully, he reached for help before pulling the trigger, and he was rescued from his tormentors. Talk therapy and some medication really helped. Overcoming the lure of a quick suicide, Pete had once again found value in living.

We talked a long time that morning. We talked about fear and courage — and how the two can work in tandem during situations like Pete faced in Vietnam. We agreed that courage is bravery in the midst of fear, and this is what he had lived through. He and his buddies had refused to surrender despite incredible fear and trepidation. They knew life would be theirs with surrender, and yet, that kind of life might be worse than death. As G. K. Chesterton wrote, "He must desire life like water and yet drink death like wine."

For one night, these soldiers had held the power to turn water into wine.

* * *

I think about Pete often, and I know he was far braver than he ever realized. His courage had shone brightly — in open warfare and in private torment. In both situations he had been brave.

But what Pete really left me with was the recognition that our healthcare system had failed him, especially regarding mental health issues. The needs of veterans were blocked by gridlocked politicians, and the pharmaceutical industry was unable to produce the miracle drug that might have helped Pete live a normal life.

Doctors had missed what Pete was enduring. I had missed his pain. In his time of critical need, there had been no support system present to help. But he battled his way out of a dark murky place. Pete became his own best champion of his health — physically, mentally, and spiritually. He won the battle so many others lost. But his journey demands that questions be asked.

How can we provide our veterans with prompt access to high quality healthcare with an emphasis on mental health needs?

How can we increase physician awareness of common post-military service issues such as PTSD, panic attacks, societal reintegration, depression, and suicide?

Is the government-run VA healthcare system the ideal way to care for veterans?

Does the VA healthcare system need support in ways not yet recognized?

Are veterans' needs getting adequate attention from those who can make a difference?

In a complicated world filled with Big Government programs, Big Pharma drugs, and Big Tech social media platforms, how can veterans like Pete find the help they need to win their toughest battles — overcoming hidden torments?

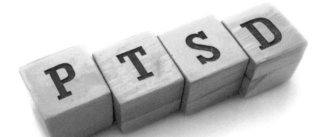

PTSD IS NOT THE PERSON REFUSING TO LET GO OF THE PAST, BUT THE PAST REFUSING TO LET GO OF THE PERSON.

—Anonymous

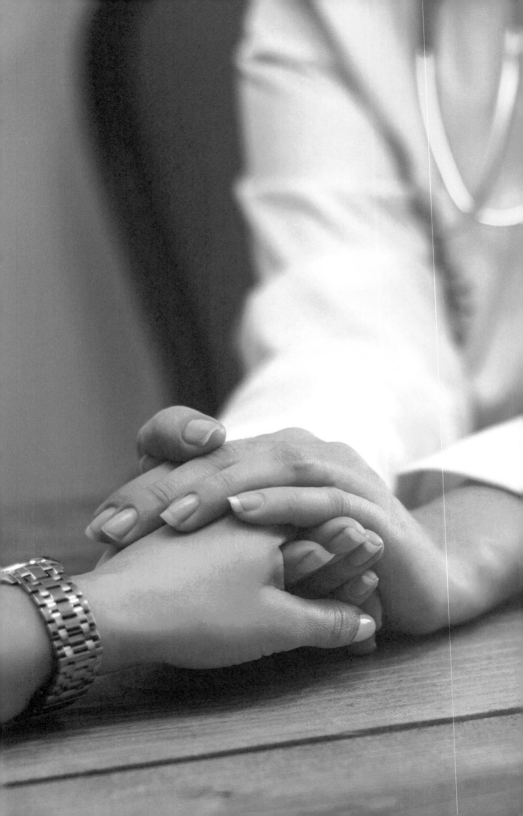

CHAPTER SIXTEEN

IS THERE A BILLING CODE FOR

COMPASSION?

Famed author and professor Leo Buscaglia once said, "Too often we underestimate the power of a touch, a smile, a kind word, a listening ear, an honest compliment, or the smallest act of caring, all of which have the potential to turn a life around." He is right, and I have seen firsthand the power of compassion unleashed to heal lives and mend hearts. Compassion is nothing less than reaching out in concern and care for the sufferings or misfortunes of others. Below is an example of what I am referring to. Nothing takes the place of compassion.

* * *

I remember a patient I saw about two years ago. She was a lady who I had privately nicknamed "Gabby Abby." Abby was one of those delightful people who brightens any room she enters. She brings sunshine with her even on rainy days, and if you happen to be feeling down when you meet her, chances are good you won't be feeling down when she leaves. But lately I had become very concerned about Abby because I knew she had suffered an intense trauma. Her husband, the love of her life, had recently died, and I wondered how she was doing at picking up the pieces of her life and moving forward.

On the day of her appointment I could see that she was clearly despondent and avoided eye contact. She wasn't herself, not by a long stretch, so I asked her, "Abby, you've been through a lot with your husband's death, and I'm concerned about you. Is there anything I can do to help?"

She started to cry, and after a few moments she slowly opened up, sharing with me that she had lost her way in terms of being with others. She felt as though half of her was missing and she didn't know what to do or who she was without her husband.

I asked her to tell me more about that. She told me about a friendship that she cherished and relied on, but somehow it had been fractured since the death of her husband. It wasn't a slow and subtle parting of the ways, but happened very abruptly. At first she wasn't sure why, but after some reflection she thought she understood what had happened. Her vital friendship was broken simply because two people didn't understand where each other was coming from. It had sent her into a tailspin and shattered her sense of self-worth. Without her husband there to reassure her that she was loved by many people, Abby felt lost. His reaffirming nature had given her more strength than she had realized, and now she was struggling. She couldn't cope. Life had changed for her. She had lost her way.

Often in situations like Abby's there are physicians who will reach for their pad and write out a prescription for Prozac, Xanax, or Trazadone. I understand that many of them think they are being compassionate by doing so, but I assure you that in many cases they are not. In fact, Abby did ask me about whether or not I thought she needed a prescription for an anti-depressant. Granted, there is a time and place for these medications, but in Abby's case I felt it was important that she try to work through the grieving process without medications. The loss of her husband had rocked her world, but she was not suicidal or emotionally "stuck." She was in need of support, and I believed I could provide that for her, at least for a while.

"Abby, the grief you're experiencing now is a normal process," I told her. "You're a strong and loving person and you'll get through this. I've seen folks who have been prescribed anti-depressants and

come to rely on them in order to cope with life. Drugs can become an impediment to the necessary process of pushing through grief. Abby, you're working through it right now, and you're doing okay."

I added, "Abby, we can't control the rhythm and events of life, but I've known you for many years, and you are strong enough to get through this. If this broken relationship with your friend can't be repaired presently, then you need to focus on other relationships and enjoy them. Keep focusing on kindness and thankfulness and expressing it whenever you can. Believe me, there are so many people who just need someone to be kind to them, to smile at them, and to talk to them. You have the God-given gifts to do these things, better than anybody I know. You'll be surprised at all the wonderful things that can happen as a result. And I'll be here any time you need me."

She smiled shyly, "I know you're right, Dr. Jensen. I guess I just needed your push. Thanks."

I saw her again a few months later. This time Abby wore a broad smile and was just as chatty as ever, without any hint of depression. She was restored and it gave me great joy to see her celebrating life and spreading her gift of cheer.

To me, the trauma that Abby had experienced was what I would refer to as "situational melancholy." Her coping skills had been temporarily crippled with the loss of her husband, and a difficult time with a friend had exacerbated her crisis. Her perceived lack of ability to endure and move forward without her husband had translated into a temporary funk. She needed a boost to get through those tough times, and I was grateful the relationship she and I shared had helped. She knew I cared and that I was there for her. I advocated for her and that helped her *trust me. Ultimately her trust turned inwards, and she began to see herself the way the rest of the world saw her — as a person of goodness.*

* * *

The cure for Abby was not a pill. It was the power of a smile, a kind word, a listening ear, an honest compliment, and the simple act of caring. These are the human gifts that helped to rescue her. That is how advocacy and trust can build on each other and produce marvelous results. When a caring person gets involved, a mind in pieces can become a mind at peace.

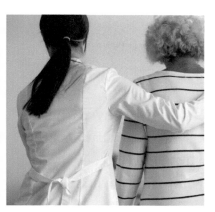

A kind word, a listening ear, an honest compliment, and the simple act of caring — these are human gifts that don't come with a billing code.

Issues to Consider

When patients are in need of support regarding acute mental health challenges brought on by emotional or physical trauma, too often physicians are inclined to prescribe anti-depressants or anti-anxiety pills or refer those patients elsewhere.

That approach makes little sense to me. How can someone the patient does not know automatically become the go-to source of care for that patient? Don't get me wrong. Therapists, psychologists, and psychiatrists are all highly trained professionals who can be of profound assistance in many situations, but relationships built on trust and advocacy truly do matter!

Roadblocks erected by insurance companies often prevent patients from having easy access to professional counseling. Navigating a mystifying labyrinth of complicated coding requirements or prior authorizations is frustrating for physicians trying to help patients through situational crises. Often insurance companies discourage doctors from getting involved with any type of mental health issues by discounting more deeply than usual physicians' charges. Too often patients are forced to make extra out-of-pocket payments for office visits if the primary diagnosis is a mental health issue.

When insurance companies decide to downgrade payments for mental health services, or restrict payment for such services to only psychiatrists or psychologists, our system of providing access to mental health services is clearly broken.

"The good physician treats the disease;

the GREAT PHYSICIAN

treats the patient who has the disease."

—William Osler

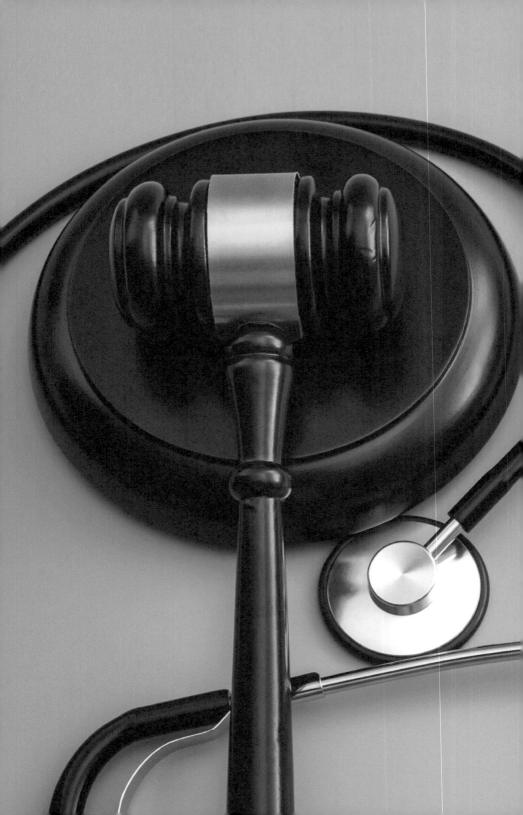

CHAPTER SEVENTEEN

A
SACRED
OATH

A patient-doctor relationship filled with candor, honesty, and sharing is no small gift. In fact, it is the very basis of a critical recycling loop: doctors advocating for patients leads to patients trusting their doctors. This repeating process of advocating and trusting creates the fertile ground from which stems high quality patient care and lasting, satisfying physician careers.

* * *

It was a cold and blustery day when I walked into the exam room and saw Mason's furrowed brow. Wasting no time I said, "Hey, Mason, what's up?"

"Doc, I don't quite know how to tell you this, but here goes. You know I get medical coverage through my wife's insurance plan where she works."

His brow was deeply furrowed and his eyes were watering, so I simply nodded in encouragement.

"Well, her employer adopted a new health insurance plan that begins the first of the year, and I won't be able to have you for my doctor anymore. Her boss says they're trying to cut costs, so they made some changes. They now have a list of pre-approved hospitals and clinics that are all part of a network that we must choose from. But your clinic is not one of our choices. So as of the first of the year we can't come to you anymore. Clare met with her boss and explained that we've been coming to you for more than a decade. Our kids weren't even walking yet. But the company made the decision, and her boss said it's totally out of his hands."

He paused before asking, "Doc, I gotta ask you, is there a reason you're not on their list of clinics?"

Frustrated, I took a deep breath and launched into a lengthy explanation.

"Mason, I understand what happened. With the onset of Obamacare the government greatly expanded its reach into the world of healthcare. Now the government is offering incentives for hospitals and clinics to form what they call Accountable Care Organizations, or ACOs. These ACOs join forces to supposedly control costs for medical services, drugs, utilization of healthcare services, and hospitalizations, among other things. If they can successfully reduce the costs of medical treatment each year for the patients who sign up under a certain plan, they are rewarded at the end of the year with increased dollars. If they don't lower costs, but instead spend too much on patients during the year, then the doctors, clinics, and hospitals may all be forced to share in covering the excess costs. In order to maximize physician output many doctors are required to reach production quotas for the number of patients they see and the charges they produce. This obviously could have an impact on the quality of care a doctor can provide, as well as patient satisfaction."

I paused a moment, then continued: "Now, to answer your question about why my clinic is not a part of that network, it's really very simple. We were not asked to join the network because we aren't a big enough player in this area. Our clinic is small and the ACOs usually look for big players who have electronic health records and a substantial internal audit capability. They also want clinics and doctors who will follow their rules and operational strategies. That is where I balk. No one is going to dictate to me or any of the doctors working at our clinics how much time we spend with our patients or what pharmacies our patients use. We're here *to serve our patients and not behemoth healthcare corporations. I decided a long time ago that I would never be a part of assembly-line medicine. I don't work on widgets. I serve patients and have taken a sacred oath. As such I do my very best with each and every patient. And let me tell you, Mason, when that oath is no longer guiding the way I care for my patients, I am done. Fact of the matter is I can think of several doctors who quit medicine simply because they would not violate the pledge they took as to how they would care for their patients.*

"I'm sorry you and your family got caught in the middle of this dehumanizing world of ACOs. But please remember, Mason, you and I have a relationship forged over time. We've enjoyed working together. You can call me anytime even if you primarily see doctors at a different clinic."

I think Mason walked out of our office that day feeling a little empty about disconnecting from our clinic. But he was also relieved that the necessary gut-wrenching discussion was over. We both shared a hope that we would reconnect in the future, and that was a balm for Mason's hurt.

* * *

Today's healthcare scene is a tough business, and without a doubt many of its component parts are broken. When patient-doctor relationships are severed for little reason other than profit and power, something is wrong.

What we are seeing today with doctors being forced to see a prescribed number of patients each day is nothing more or less than assembly-line medicine. It not only impacts the quality of healthcare that can be provided, but it also creates other issues that may have long term consequences detrimental to the patients.

For example, the opioid crisis is directly related to the over-prescribing of "pain killers," which has in part been caused by doctors and clinics with limited time relying on Big Pharma to help them lessen the suffering of their patients. At one point opioids were indiscriminately over-prescribed at the recommendation of the large pharmaceutical companies and with the false assurance of no likely addictive issues. Doctors did wrong. And when the death toll started to tick upwards, physicians did not want to wear the mantle of guilt. But their culpability was apparent, and now the system of how patients are cared for needs to be analyzed and improved.

The American healthcare system is broken, and government, insurance companies, and Big Pharma seem to be in no great hurry to fix it.

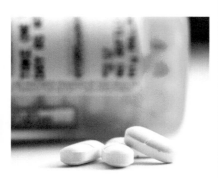

When patient-doctor relationships are severed for little reason other than profit and power, something is wrong.

Issues to Ponder

When government incentivizes clinics, hospitals, mega-pharmacies, and insurance companies to form large corporations, it should be no great surprise that such monster organizations might disrupt established relationships between patient and doctor, patient and pharmacist, patient and hospital, and many other patient-based bonds. This kind of influence in healthcare creates many unfortunate and unintended consequences.

How can we as a society preserve what truly makes for the best healthcare — quality, trusted relationships — while understanding that inflation of utilization and cost in our healthcare system has to be addressed?

When patients are forced to give up trusted connecting points to quality medical care, they quickly learn that they are not at the center of our healthcare system. When they are relegated to the role of a mere unit in a business model, they are then ripe for feelings of loss and loneliness that give birth to out-of-control anxiety, depression, and suicidal thoughts.

Do potential increased profits for a newly founded Accountable Care Organization justify turning the medical care of patients inside out?

Should smaller physician clinics be disallowed from joining larger networks just because of size?

Should "any willing provider" legislation be approved so that doctors willing to abide by an insurance company's rules be allowed to see that company's insured patients?

Is it acceptable for insurance companies, government agencies, and ACOs to mandate that patients only be allowed to go to clinics and hospitals on an "approved" list?

When clinics, hospitals, mega-pharmacies, and insurance companies form large corporations, is there a conflict of interest for a physician to be rewarded financially if he or she can reduce the amount of services provided, and dollars spent, for patients?

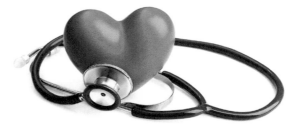

Doctor-patient relationship is part of the HEALING PROCESS.

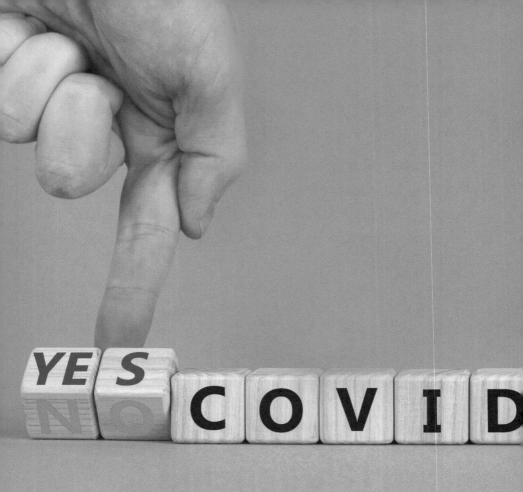

CHAPTER EIGHTEEN

Should I or Shouldn't I?

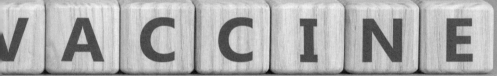

Over the past four decades as a practicing physician, I have cared for hundreds of thousands of patients with scores of varying healthcare needs. But never has the challenge of advising patients been as intense for me — or countless other physicians — as during the COVID pandemic. I anticipate that my future as a physician will be filled with such nagging personal questions as: Who drove us to such fear? What could I have done differently? How could the COVID crisis have generated such an intense and lasting drama of division, conflict, and rancor among my own fraternity of otherwise kind, compassionate, and fair-minded medical professionals?

Throughout the heat of the COVID pandemic my practice was constantly impacted by new patients arriving along with many long-established patients departing. For most of these patients, their reasons for coming or going had nothing to do with the care they received. Instead, it was all about the "elephant in the room" — meaning, what I thought about COVID and all the issues surrounding it: lockdowns, closures, masks, vaccines, vaccine mandates and passports, boosters, hydroxychloroquine, ivermectin, and whatever else the sensation-driven media considered news at any given moment.

Throughout this entire ordeal, the most agonizing topic for my patients was whether or not they should get the COVID vaccine in one of its various forms. While the breadth of perspectives on this issue is critically important, a deep dive into this heated topic is beyond the scope of a book striving to shine a bright light on our broken U.S. healthcare system, and how we can return it to its original goal of providing a path to healing and health for individuals and families.

Suffice it to say that our current method of caring for people has proven to be woefully inadequate. The traditional trust-based relationship between healer and patient has been fractured. Confidence in public health officials can no longer be assumed, and this will undoubtedly impact the willingness of citizens to abide by future public health edicts or recommendations. The nature of the recent COVID vaccine campaign revealed the terrifying truth that when Big Pharma, Big Tech, and Big Government join forces to accomplish a shared agenda, patients may suffer and voices may be cancelled.

As I interacted with my patients throughout the COVID pandemic, I routinely encountered "vaccine hesitancy," an uncertainty regarding the scientific establishment of safety and/or efficacy of the COVID vaccines. These patients were not 'conspiracy theorists.' They simply had some vaccine concerns, informed consent issues, and saw the deep national divide as further evidence that all that needed to be known about the vaccines was not yet known. Many of these folks also had a deep-seated belief that they were entitled to absolute health freedom, a right protected by the Constitution.

It is important to understand that this phenomenon of 'vaccine hesitancy' is not something new. It has been around for decades. In fact, a glimpse into my visit with a patient I'll call Darlene might help build a bridge of understanding regarding the challenges many people face concerning vaccine decision-making in an era of emerging pandemics like COVID.

* * *

"Doctor Jensen, I just don't know!" Darlene began one day in my office. "Should I get the COVID vaccine or not? I guess I understand

that it's a personal decision, but I'm really nervous about getting the vaccine because it seems like such a rush job. And yet the possibility of putting this darned pandemic behind us sort of makes me want to go for it and get it over with.

"But then I watch the news and, gee whiz, the sales pitch is so over the top that I wonder why government officials are pushing so hard! And honestly, Doctor, I'm not a conspiracy kind of person, but I feel so helpless! I find myself getting angry at some of the off-the-wall 'experts' who come out with crazy ideas like the government using the vaccine to track me and — I'm sure you've heard some of these wacky ideas! My anxiety level is off the charts!

"And then from the other side I hear, 'Do your part! Herd immunity is just around the corner. Get your vaccine passport and start living again — yada, yada, yada.

"At the end of it all what I keep coming back to is this: I'm in good health and I don't take flu shots. I don't like taking pills, and I don't like the idea of injecting anything into my body. I remember well what Dr. Fauci said about a vaccine normally taking years to be developed and certainly couldn't happen in less than 12 to 18 months. But they rolled these vaccines out in months and pushed everyone to get them immediately and shamed anyone who expressed concerns. Something just isn't right! Can you please tell me what to do?"

After a moment to let all she said sink in, I responded: "Darlene, I can't tell you what to do. You might reasonably compare a COVID vaccination to an annual flu shot. You might figure that you're healthy and COVID would present little challenge to you. But then, you're seventy years old. And you have complained about not being able to be with your grandkids. You like to travel, and your *husband is definitely vulnerable. You're old enough to remember how some vaccines saved millions of lives. These are all important considerations. If you were twenty-five years old with different circumstances, I might be telling you that getting COVID would not likely be a serious issue for you and that the notion of a societal obligation to take the vaccine may not be the ideal basis for your decision. I don't mean to be evasive, but the fact of the matter is that there's no one right answer for everyone. I'm sorry that I can't be more definitive, but these are uncharted waters we are navigating."*

I continued: "Darlene, it's important to realize that COVID vaccines provide vulnerable folks a better chance to avoid hospitalization or death, but they don't completely eliminate these potentialities. What I am telling you, Darlene, is that thousands of vaccinated and vulnerable patients will still get the disease, and some will die. It's no fun telling folks that the vaccines aren't perfect cure-alls, but it needs to be said. For me that's part and parcel of true 'informed consent.'

"While the news media has dishonestly portrayed me as being against the vaccines, the truth is that I am simply for the freedom of you and all my patients to make your own choice. And that has been my firm conviction for over forty years of practicing medicine.

"So my best suggestion, Darlene, is to do your homework and make your own decision. But remember, there is no one correct decision. One size does not fit all when it comes to medical decisions."

Concluding our appointment, I assured Darlene that whatever decision she made, I would be there for her and would continue to support her. "I feel your frustration about not knowing what to do," I said. "Lots of folks will tell you not to make a big deal out of it and go ahead and get the vaccine. Others will say the opposite. But one thing you might not hear is the simple fact that you can't get unvaccinated. Through the years involving a variety of vaccines, I have had numerous gut-wrenching conversations with folks who got vaccinated and then had second thoughts about whether they did the right thing. That's what makes this so difficult. But whatever you decide, I'm here for you."

As I exited the exam room, I had the sinking feeling that I hadn't really helped Darlene with her tough question: "Should I or shouldn't I . . ."

* * *

Trying to provide patients with the information necessary to meet the vague criteria for what qualifies as "informed consent" is an ever-present challenge for doctors. In Darlene's situation there was so much more I could have said. The following information may have been helpful for her, but I worried it would simply overwhelm an already fragile patient who wanted to take the easy way out by having me decide for her.

How much to say is always a judgement call, and I am certain I occasionally miss the mark. The following concerns are not a part of my routine patient discussion, but they do form the basis for my own personal skepticism regarding so many public policy decisions made throughout the COVID pandemic:

- Blatant profiteering by Big Pharma and others during the pandemic.

- Unprecedented public health/government overreach into the private lives of citizens.

- The role of Big Tech and the major media in cancelling opposing voices.

- The betrayal and abandonment of patients by doctors and healthcare players.

- Ethical lapses by Big Pharma.

- The monopolization by Big Tech of the information and opinions to which people are allowed access.

- The lack of high-quality human data establishing the short- and long-term safety and effectiveness of the COVID vaccines.

- The over-emphasis by insurance conglomerates on gross revenues.

- The questionable sales tactics of medical vendors.

- The use of personal attacks by politicians, bureaucrats, and physicians toward those with differing perspectives on COVID strategies and policies.

- The minimization of Vaccine Adverse Event Reporting System (VAERS) data and its importance in analyzing the pros and cons of the various COVID vaccines.

- The willingness of public health officials to disregard the potential value of natural immunity for COVID.

- The use of unethical and immoral vaccine passport policies.

- The willingness of government officials to impose lockdown policies resulting in devastating collateral damage.

- The lack of integrity on the part of fact checkers.

Throughout the pandemic, millions of Americans felt like they were "being played" — often via a Big Government agenda that intersected too conveniently with Big Tech interests and Big Pharma revenues. Throughout the many tortuous months of living under a hovering COVID cloud, I advocated for an understanding based on context and shaped by seeing events through a new lens, a lens that exposes powerful stakeholders for what they are and what they do. The treacherous threesome — Big Government, Big Tech, and Big Pharma — has accumulated a long list of sins, and the price of such transgressions has yet to be determined.

The bottom line in all of this is that patients must have real freedom in making decisions about matters of their own health. Trusting a system to stand for individual health freedom is an oxymoron. Despite what the "experts" say, every patient must have the right to choose the interventions he or she utilizes and the privilege to determine how personal healthcare will be pursued.

As a physician I have appreciated how vaccines prevent and mitigate disease. Indeed, I spend several hundred thousand dollars every year on various vaccines for my patients. As for COVID, data reveals that patients over 70 years of age with underlying medical conditions have a one-in-twenty chance of dying from COVID without the vaccine, but a less than one-in-twenty thousand chance of dying from the COVID vaccine (if they opt to take the vaccine). That data is a big part of the reason more than 95 percent of my patients over 70 years of age have chosen to be vaccinated against COVID.

Nonetheless, the very thought of forcing my patients to take a vaccination violates every fiber of who I am. I will honor their choices as I have for forty years. I will advocate for my patients, and in so doing it is my hope that they will come to trust me.

Most importantly, it is my goal to be a part of the motivating forces by which patients are encouraged and empowered to be their own best healthcare champions.

For my patients, I will always stand for health freedom.

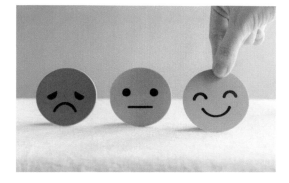

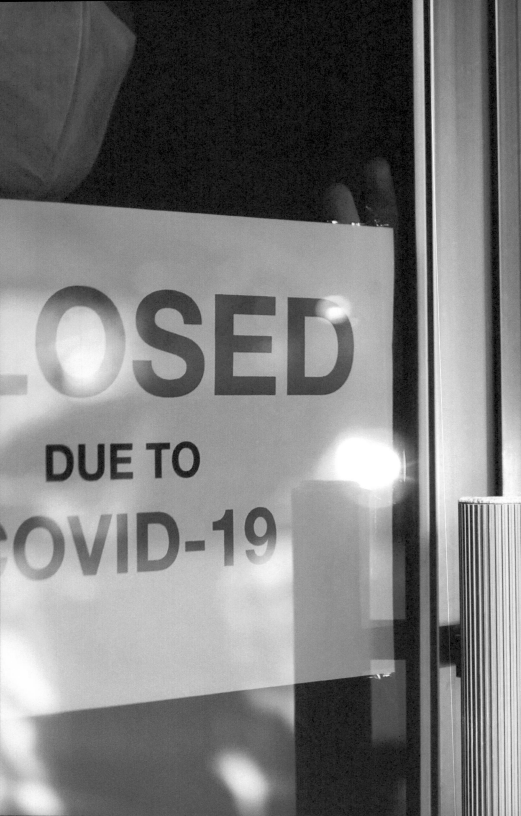

CHAPTER NINETEEN

LOCKDOWNS:

WHEN THE WORLD WENT MAD

"To the future or to the past, to a time when thought is free ... to a time when truth exists and what is done cannot be undone ... greetings!"
—George Orwell, *1984*

I was in high school when our class read George Orwell's dystopian novel, *1984*. It generated a great deal of heated discussion that ran the gamut from one extreme to the other. Some said that the world Orwell predicted could never happen, while others felt that it was already occurring, little by little, without our really even knowing it. I leaned toward the opinion that, because we lived in America, we were immune to such an awful nightmare. It simply could never happen here.

It wasn't until a few years ago when I saw the movie series, *The Hunger Games*, that I began to ruminate on the notion that Orwell's *1984* prediction might indeed be far more than mere fantasy.

Then came March 2020. It seemed like the world was going mad as our nation and the rest of the earth went into an extended "lockdown." Suddenly *The Hunger Games* and *1984* were never far from my mind. Sheltering in place and rigid edicts became the government's new *modus operandi*. Businesses were shuttered, restaurants, schools, and churches were closed, concerts and sporting events were cancelled, mask mandates and social distancing dictates were implemented. The erosion of our freedoms became commonplace — and truly, the scenario of

1984 was upon us.

Nearly overnight the constitutionally guaranteed rights of Americans were suspended, due process was thrown out, free speech was curtailed, and the right to peaceably assemble was retracted. Big Tech piled on by applying the heavy hand of censorship and cancellation whenever and wherever it chose. A government takedown was perpetrated under the guise of a panic-driven pandemic.

Lost in the chaos was the bedrock understanding that our individual rights, guaranteed by the U.S. Constitution, are granted by God, not man. The purpose of civil government is to protect and preserve those rights. Government is not their originator, and as such, nowhere in the Constitution or in any of our founding documents does it say those rights can be suspended or removed because of some proclamation from a bureaucrat or politician, regardless of perceived calamity or crisis. Elected officials are tasked with the responsibility to promote the "general welfare," but not under the proviso of trampling underfoot all the other rights they have a sworn duty to uphold.

The Hunger Games took on a whole new level of disturbing relevance when Supreme Court Justice Samuel Alito made the following comments in November 2020:

> *The pandemic has resulted in previously unimaginable restrictions on individual liberty ... it is an indisputable statement of fact. We have never before seen restrictions as severe, extensive and prolonged as those experienced for most of 2020. Think of all the live events that would otherwise be protected by the right to freedom of speech, live speeches, conferences, lectures, meetings. Think of*

worship services. Churches closed on Easter Sunday, synagogues closed for Passover and Yom Kippur. Think about access to the courts or the constitutional right to a speedy trial. Who could have imagined that? The COVID crisis has served as a sort of constitutional stress test and in doing so, it has highlighted disturbing trends that were already present before the virus struck.

Indeed, we had been thrust into a bizarre new world order where dystopian fears no longer seem unimaginable.

* * *

When It's Time to Speak Up

My cellphone rang and I did not recognize the number of the caller. I hesitated, thinking it might be another one of those unwanted sales calls, but decided to answer it anyway. "Hello, Scott Jensen here."

There was a brief pause and then a voice almost cracking with emotion: "Dr. Jensen, you don't know me, but I know you through social media and the news. I just had to call you."

I had no idea what was going to come next, but I was touched by the raw sadness her voice conveyed.

"Dr. Jensen, I'm a physician also, but I'm really struggling — struggling to find courage like you have. I feel terrible that you're standing alone. I just wish I could do what you've been doing. But I have so much to risk, and yet I know I should be speaking up."

There was a long pause, so I offered, "Well, thank you. I appreciate your words very much."

She blurted haltingly, "If I say anything publicly, it will mean getting investigated by the Board of Medical Practice, and I don't want to lose my job. I can't. I have bills to pay. I know that's no excuse, but ... "

I had no ready words to soothe her anxiety.

She continued, "I notice that you signed the 'Great Barrington Declaration.'"

"Yes, I did," I responded quietly.

"It's an impressive document," she said, followed by another long pause, then, "Thank you for signing it. I thought about doing the same, but..."

There was more awkward silence, so I volunteered, "I didn't get your name."

"Carole."

"Carole, I understand where you're coming from. Putting your name on something can have downstream consequences you could never expect. I signed it because it absolutely reflects my views, especially in regards to the many ill-conceived policies our state department of health has instituted. It also recognizes the fact that our constitutional rights have been short-circuited, and that's really important to me. In fact, when I finished reading it, I really didn't have much choice but to sign it right away."

I chose my next words cautiously: "Carole, I think I understand the situation you're in. Not everybody has the same latitude in how to respond to these bizarre times. We've all got to figure out our own unique path."

"Thank you, Dr. Jensen. Those words are kind. I appreciate your compassion. I've taken enough of your time. I hope someday we can meet in person."

A Document Worth Defending

So what exactly is the "Great Barrington Declaration"? It is a statement written by three public health experts from Harvard, Stanford, and Oxford, encouraging governments to lift lockdown restrictions on young and healthy people, while focusing protection measures on the elderly. They note that the restrictions posed by lockdown have caused vast collateral harm, including lower childhood vaccination rates, worsening cardiovascular disease outcomes, fewer cancer screenings, and dramatic increases in mental health crises, not to mention a record-setting increase in drug overdose deaths. The "Great Barrington Declaration" is crafted with care and precision. It gave me great satisfaction to sign it promptly, and I share it below.

* * *

On October 4, 2020, the **Great Barrington Declaration** was authored and signed in Great Barrington, Massachusetts, by:

Dr. Martin Kulldorff, professor of medicine at Harvard University, a biostatistician, and epidemiologist with expertise in detecting and monitoring infectious disease outbreaks and vaccine safety evaluations.

Dr. Sunetra Gupta, professor at Oxford University, an epidemiologist with expertise in immunology, vaccine development, and mathematical modeling of infectious diseases.

Dr. Jay Bhattacharya, professor at Stanford University Medical School, a physician, epidemiologist, health economist, and public health policy expert focusing on infectious diseases and vulnerable populations.

The Great Barrington Declaration

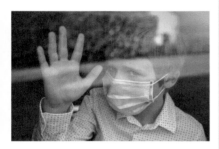

We have been thrust into an unfinished chapter of some brave new world, where our dystopian fears no longer seem so unimaginable. It is time for us to wake up and take action!

As infectious disease epidemiologists and public health scientists we have grave concerns about the damaging physical and mental health impacts of the prevailing COVID-19 policies, and recommend an approach we call Focused Protection.

Coming from both the left and right, and around the world, we have devoted our careers to protecting people. Current lockdown policies are producing devastating effects on short and long-term public health. The results (to name a few) include lower childhood vaccination rates, worsening cardiovascular disease outcomes, fewer cancer screenings and deteriorating mental health — leading to greater excess mortality in years to come, with the working class and younger members of society carrying the heaviest burden. Keeping students out of school is a grave injustice.

Keeping these measures in place until a vaccine is available will cause irreparable damage, with the underprivileged disproportionately harmed.

Fortunately, our understanding of the virus is growing. We know that vulnerability to death from COVID-19 is more than a thousand-fold higher in the old and infirm than the young. Indeed, for children, COVID-19 is less dangerous than many other harms including influenza.

As immunity builds in the population, the risk of infection to all — including the vulnerable — falls. We know that all populations will eventually reach herd immunity — i.e. the point at which the rate of new infections is stable — and that this can be assisted by (but is not dependent upon) a vaccine. Our goal should therefore be to minimize mortality and social harm until we reach herd immunity.

The most compassionate approach that balances the risks and benefits of reaching herd immunity is to allow those who are at minimal risk of death to live their lives normally to build up immunity to the virus through natural infection, while better protecting those who are at highest risk. We call this Focused Protection.

Adopting measures to protect the vulnerable should be the central aim of public health responses to COVID-19. By way of example, nursing homes should use staff with acquired immunity and perform frequent testing of other staff and all visitors. Staff rotation should be minimized. Retired people living at home should have groceries and other essentials delivered to their home. When possible, they should meet family members outside rather than inside. A comprehensive and detailed list of measures, including approaches to multi-generational households, can be implemented, and is well within the scope and capability of public health professionals.

Those who are not vulnerable should immediately be allowed to resume life as normal. Simple hygiene measures, such as hand washing and staying home when sick should be practiced by everyone to reduce the herd immunity threshold. Schools and universities should be open for in-person teaching. Extracurricular activities, such as sports, should be resumed. Young low-risk adults should work normally, rather than from home. Restaurants and other businesses should open. Arts, music, sports, and other cultural activities should resume. People who are more at risk may participate if they wish, while society as a whole enjoys the protection conferred upon the vulnerable by those who have built up herd immunity.

IF THE GOVERNMENT CAN SUSPEND YOUR RIGHTS ANYTIME IT SEES FIT, YOU DON'T HAVE RIGHTS. YOU HAVE PRIVILEGES.

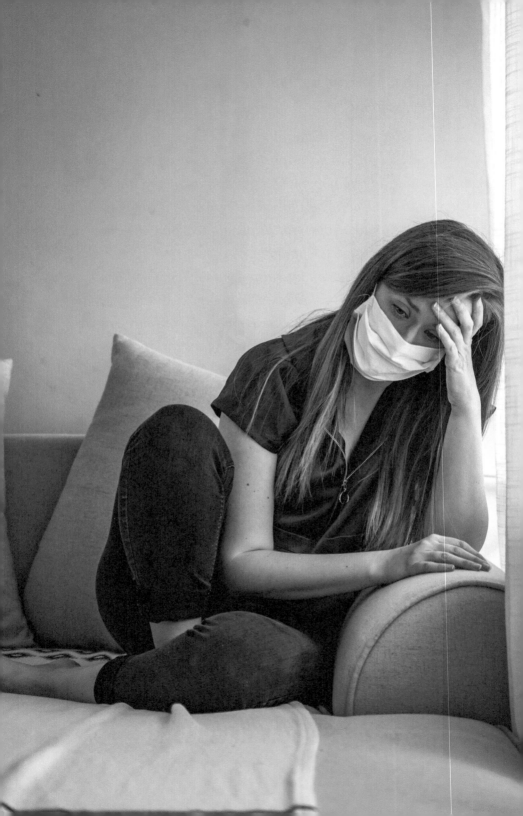

CHAPTER TWENTY

SACRIFICING SCIENCE
on the ALTAR of
F.E.A.R.

Billy was shaking. A tough blue-collar worker not frightened by much was panicked. A thirty-year-old father of two kids, married to a delightful and optimistic wife, was petrified by fear. Why? How? Unfortunately, Billy's visit to my medical clinic was prompted by an all too common phenomenon — fear of COVID and fear of what COVID was causing all of us to become. Billy's voice quivered, "Doctor Jensen, what in the world is going on?"

In an ideal situation I would have told Billy that we all face fears of different kinds, and we have to deal with those fears in a variety of ways. It is a part of the experience we call being human. Fear can come in an instant and throw us into chaos, yet it can also save our lives. Fear is a natural response to real physical danger, or a perceived threat, whether real or imagined. It comes to us in many forms. It can be self-generated, such as the fear of failure, the fear of being out of control, the fear of being different, or even the fear of being lonely. There is also fear of the future and of death. Some people even fear love, because they fear being rejected. Others become miserly because they fear they won't have enough. Still others struggle to share their feelings or have difficulty trusting, because they are dominated by self-doubt and insecurity, or are afraid of being wrong.

These fears are normal and common to all of us. The good news is that as we grow and mature as individuals, when we face these fears head-on and overcome them, we are stronger for them. That is a natural part of life and growing up.

But there is another kind of fear that is not good, one that is far more insidious and destructive, one that, if left unchallenged and unchecked, will destroy the lives and livelihoods of millions of people and perhaps even our nation. It is a fear that has been utterly fabricated, projected upon the unsuspecting masses, and turned into an abhorrent expected sacrifice that is destroying the foundation of all that we hold dear. That is F.E.A.R. — or False Evidence Appearing Real.

F.E.A.R. is the poisonous fruit of a false narrative. History can tell us just how powerful well-crafted false narratives or lies can be. They have been used hundreds of times to create panic and a sense of helplessness in the masses. When masterfully fashioned, they can be diabolically effective. They have been used to start wars, divide kingdoms, and crash economies. When told well, they are convincing. Nothing will make the masses more compliant and so easily manipulated as a narrative that keeps them rooted in perpetual fear. We have seen this played out before our very eyes as the driving force of the COVID-19 pandemic.

In February 2020 I was taken by surprise and blindsided, as were millions of my medical colleagues worldwide, when it was reported that a tremendously contagious virus with extremely lethal characteristics was emerging on the world scene from the province of Wuhan, China. Alarming videos were splashed all over TV and aggressively forwarded to social media platforms showing Chinese people dying, hospitals overrun, and non-compliant folks being rounded up by police in hazmat suits. To say it was frightening is an understatement. Early reports warned that Europe and the U.S. were both in the crosshairs of this lethal virus that was spreading like wildfire.

The initial information was sketchy at best, but it wasn't long before this virus was being compared to the infamous Spanish flu pandemic of 1918-1920, that resulted in over 50 million deaths worldwide, with at least 675,000 deaths occurring in the U.S. alone. With the world population at 7.8 billion today — four times what it was in 1918 — some models projected a potential death toll as high as 200 million for this COVID pandemic! The U.S. was projected to witness as many as 2.5 million deaths.

There was little information regarding specific methods and protocols for treating COVID, so it wasn't difficult to understand why doctors worldwide were willing to cooperate with the restrictive protocols and societal controls that were immediately put in place. With COVID-19 threatening to become a global pandemic of unprecedented magnitude, bureaucrats insisted that the only logical and reasonable step was for the entire planet to cooperate in a worldwide lockdown to stem its spread.

With the lockdown came the cessation of public meetings, along with the closing of businesses and places where people congregated such as restaurants, theaters, clubs, stadiums, gyms, hair salons, and even churches — all in the hope of minimizing exposure and possible transmission of the virus.

People were to stay at home, and only the most essential workers were allowed to be outside, and only then to go directly to and from their jobs. Schools were closed for in-person classes, and distance online learning became the norm. Curfews were imposed. The media constantly reported on the growth and expansion of the virus, keeping a daily tally of cases/infections and a running death count.

Never in all of history had such an effective ploy been used to keep the populations of the earth stuck in perpetual F.E.A.R. Never had we quarantined the healthy to supposedly protect those in most danger — the frail and weak. Never had we convinced the world that a pandemic could be spread through asymptomatic people. We turned healthy individuals into walking, talking potential threats. Concerts, public gatherings, beach outings, and even church choir practices were all banned, for fear that they might become "super-spreader" events. Any gatherings of more than ten people were halted, and even having friends over to your house was strongly discouraged. Thus, we needed to isolate and stay away from one another because of the virulence of the invisible threat. Added to it all was the utter necessity of everyone using a face covering, even when inside, even when eating, only to be removed in between bites.

There was a worldwide scramble for Personal Protective Equipment — gloves, masks, gowns, and shields. Businesses installed plexiglass barriers to keep people as separated as possible during transactions. Everyone was to constantly wash their hands. Hand sanitizer was an essential for every home, every business, every person. Social distancing was implemented, with a required minimum distance of six feet between every human. Hugs were dangerous, and shaking hands was forbidden. The virus could be anywhere and everywhere. No one and nowhere was safe. Toilet paper was hoarded, and cereal boxes were sterilized before stored in the cupboard.

Did the sky fall? No. Did all the fear-filled prognostications come true? Of course not! Is the virus real? Yes. Is it as dangerous and awful as it has been promoted to be? For the bulk of the population, not at all. For the elderly or those with co-morbidities, it certainly can be serious. It is no trifling matter.

Yet, even if it is dangerous for a small segment, according to the CDC, the vast majority of people will experience an encouraging survivability rate for COVID-19 as follows:

0-19 years	99.997%
20-49 years	99.98%
50-69 years	99.5%
70+ higher	94.6%

As more information and true evidence-based science has come to light, the danger of COVID-19 appears to stem more from the policies and agenda of fear than from any actual medical realities. The fact that some horrible mistakes were made leading to the needless deaths of thousands only exacerbated the situation.

The health and well-being of the individual patient was sacrificed at the altar of fear because public health officials failed to first diagnose the problem correctly. Horrific assumptions were made, and many of these proved deadly.

In all humility, there is much that we still do not know. So anyone making hard and fast declarations about all this is not acting in wisdom. That said, every day more and more information is coming forth that is causing us to challenge the wisdom of the policies chosen, and even the veracity of what we had been told. That is disturbing, beyond words.

What is clear is that being governed by fear led to disaster, and made things far worse.

As always, the antidote to fear is truth. Exaggeration will not help. It will lead to wrong actions and bad policies with potentially tragic results. We need skepticism, scientific discourse, and argumentation. Good, bad or ugly, what we don't need is to be deluged with terror.

We would do well to heed the words of 20th century writer H.L. Mencken, who observed: "The urge to save humanity is almost always only a false-face for the urge to rule it. Power is what all messiahs really seek, not the chance to serve."

Pandemic projections, PCR testing, contact tracing, asymptomatic spread, and the pandemic of the unvaccinated all proved to be tools of fear-mongering.

Billy, the answer to your question, "What in the world is going on?" is this: F.E.A.R. — False Evidence Appearing Real.

But, Billy, the real question is this: Why in the world is this F.E.A.R. happening?

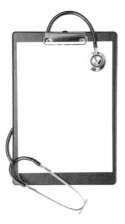

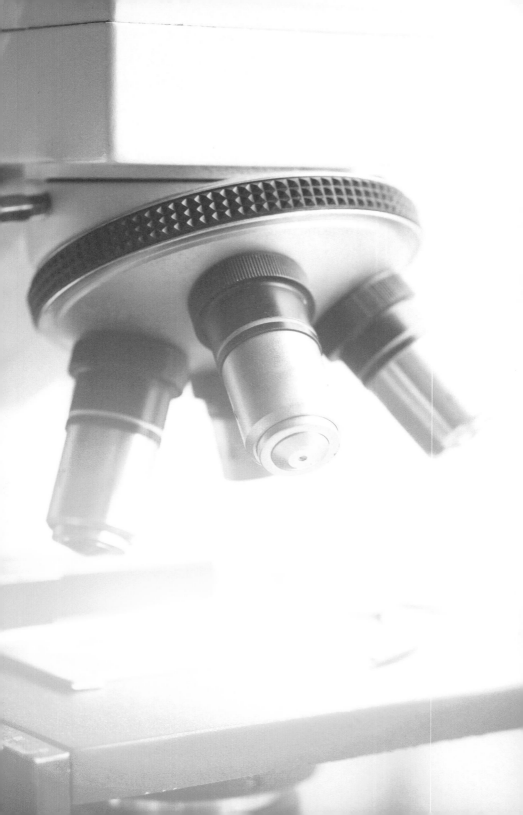

CHAPTER TWENTY ONE

OUR SIN

of Not Recognizing Science

It was mid-June of 2021, fifteen months into the pandemic. My next appointment was not so much a clinic visit with a patient. It was more of a chance to have a discussion with a friend, a nurse I had known for more than a decade. Olivia and her family had been coming to our clinic since her kids were little, and now they were nearly teenagers. Over the years, she and I had enjoyed many thought-provoking conversations, pulling back the curtain on the state of healthcare and discussing trends. And while I wasn't sure what specifically had given rise to today's appointment, I assumed our conversation would be no different than many before.

"This whole thing just feels slimy," Olivia said.

I smiled and shook my head. Strong opinions and plain talk were Olivia's specialty. Taking the bait, I egged her on. "Okay, Olivia, I'll bite. What 'whole thing' are we referring to?"

"Truth is, Scott, I've got a bunch of things swirling around in my mind and I need someone I can bounce some things off of. I guess you're it. Are you game?" she asked.

"I'm not sure what I'm getting myself into," I responded, "but why not? What's our starting point?"

Her eyes sparkled, and with an impish grin she said, "Let's see, with such a target-rich environment, I hardly know where to begin."

I smiled and waited to see where she would go with this conversation.

Olivia continued: "We could ponder the wisdom of mass vaccinating the entire planet with a never-been-used-before mRNA

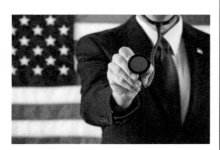

Our biggest sin is not just that we are not following the science. It is that we have forgotten how to even recognize science.

product that included shortcuts in completing animal and human safety trials. Or we could talk about what we've done to our society with these 'maskination' policies that have about as little consistency as anyone could imagine. I've always enjoyed trying to capture tiny micro-particles, invisible to the naked eye, with a piece of porous cloth."

I laughed. Olivia was on a roll.

"We do live in bizarre times, don't we?" I said. And then as an afterthought, I muttered, "It seems like somewhere along the way we lost the ability to recognize science, let alone follow it."

She nodded and said quietly, "Doctor, I really am bothered by this whole big push to vaccinate our kids! You know I'm not 'anti-vax.' And I know you're not either. You've given vaccines to my kids for decades when we thought they were appropriate. Heck, I bet you spend thousands of dollars every year for vaccines for your patients. I am so tired of the labels 'anti-vax' and 'vaccine *hesitant.' While I am for sure not anti-vax, I am anti-vaccine mandate. Government cannot coerce people. By law they must provide informed consent — real informed consent. And now the government is trying to vaccinate our kids without parental consent! What is that all about? Since when did we lose our rights as parents? Honestly, this feels like a totalitarian police state."*

"I hear you, Olivia," I answered. "You'll get no disagreement from me."

"Well, let me just say this, Doc! Over my dead body! I'm not going along with any of this."

And our discussion was over.

* * *

That was Olivia! Never subtle, never quiet. And I understood her outrage. I had my own, especially when I read what Dr. Roger Hodkinson, a renowned pathologist said about the pandemic:

[this] is politicians playing medicine, and that's an extremely dangerous game. They should stick to their knitting! They know nothing about this. It's massive deception. The lies upon lies upon lies knows no end....

I agreed wholeheartedly, and my spirit of skepticism had been bolstered. Too often "Follow the Science" has been the mantra used to bludgeon dissent — but that's exactly what we have not been doing. Our biggest sin is not just that we are not following the science. It is that we have forgotten how to even recognize science.

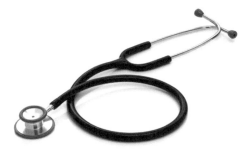

"It is hard to imagine a more stupid or more dangerous way of making decisions than by putting those decisions in the hands of people who pay no price for being wrong."

—Thomas Sowell

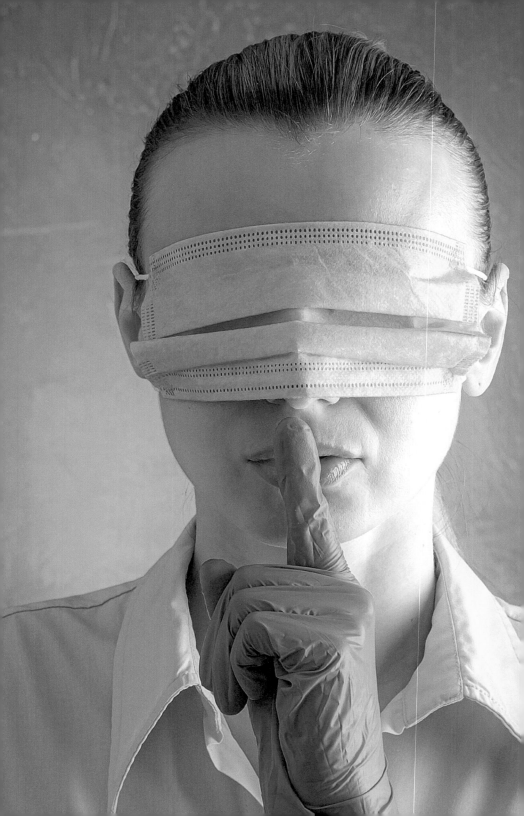

CHAPTER TWENTY TWO

BLINDED

BY OUR OWN NORMALCY BIAS

"There are none so blind as those who will not see. The most deluded people are those who choose to ignore what they already know."
— John Heywood

I stepped into the exam room and could not help but smile when I realized that the patient waiting for me was one of my all-time favorites. Nancy was simply one of the most wholesome, good-hearted individuals I had ever met. I doubt that she had ever said anything bad about anyone, ever. When she did have something to say about someone, it was always kind and good, and she meant it for the best. It was nice just to be around her. But the troubled look on her face this morning said plainly that there was something wrong.

"Nancy, is everything OK?" I asked.

Visibly disturbed and uncharacteristically terse, she snapped, "No, it's not. I don't know who and what to believe anymore."

I knew what was coming next, so I cut to the chase. "You're frustrated with all the COVID stuff aren't you?"

"Exactly!" she said. "I read the newspapers, and they say the number of cases are dropping, the death rate is going down, and there are fewer hospitalizations. But I turn on the TV and they're saying the virus is mutating, dark days are coming, and I should be more frightened than ever because the variants are going to be more deadly. Well, which is it?"

Before I could respond, Nancy continued venting, "They said '15 days to flatten the curve', and here we are two years later and none of the modeling they scared us with has happened. I know people who have gotten sick and some that have even died, but these lockdowns are ridiculous. They've shut down the entire world, and for what? They haven't stopped anything. Other nations have remained completely open, and they seem to have fared far better. The only thing they've done is destroyed my husband's business, and millions of other small businesses.

"Our children have struggled, with schools closed for an entire year, and they've forced everyone to wear these stupid masks! I can't visit my dad in the nursing home. And what they did in the nursing homes is criminal! Why in the world would you ever force nursing homes to re-admit sick people without first checking to make sure they weren't still contagious? What they did only led to more deaths. That's unconscionable! Everyone's supposed to get tested, but the PCR tests are unreliable and in short supply. Then we get scolded for clogging the emergency rooms! Why is no one doing anything to stop this?

"Now the government is basically forcing the 'vaccine' on us — spending a billion dollars in marketing, offering donuts, beer, lottery tickets. Really? If this was a real pandemic and the shot worked, would you need to convince people or bribe them to take it? All for a 'vaccine' that has no guarantee that it will prevent infection or stop transmission. Is it really 'safe and effective' — really? Then why all the reports of injury and death for those who've taken it? Jim and I both got COVID, and we both got over it. So shouldn't we have the antibodies and natural immunity? The kids never seemed to be impacted. None of this makes sense. I just want life to go back to normal!"

Nancy choked out a breath as her eyes brimmed with tears. She was surprised at her own outburst. "I'm sorry, Dr. Jensen. I'm not usually this worked up, but I am so confused and I feel so powerless to stop any of it. What is going on?"

"Nancy, don't be sorry," I replied. "I'm upset as well. I wish I could tell you what's going on, but I don't know. I don't have the answers, but I do ask the same questions."

My confession came as a definite disappointment to her, but it was the truth.

So, I continued, "I share your frustration. These constant contradictions in policy directives from our so-called 'health professionals' don't make sense. They tell us to follow the science, but there is no science to back up their policies. I can't help but wonder if there is a limit to how much Big Tech can censor contrarian voices and legitimate concerns of respected doctors worldwide who are raising critical questions that need to be heard. We need more scientific debate, not less. Why are we ignoring potentially helpful therapies that are inexpensive and readily available? Patients and doctors have always been able to mutually decide if the 'off-label' use of a medicine is something that is advisable. That's what doctors did in 1976 with the Legionnaire's pneumonia outbreak. Trust me, Nancy, doctors are confused as well. I've never seen anything like this."

While it was getting me a little riled up, Nancy found my angst strangely comforting. "So, I'm not losing my mind?" she asked.

"No, Nancy. You and millions of others are right to be concerned and to ask questions. I pride myself in being a reasonable person. I'm not into conspiracies. I'm wired to believe

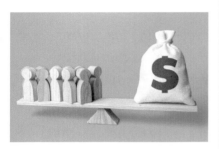

Could we choose to amend the rules of the game to create a society that values people over profits?

the best about people. I tend to give them the benefit of the doubt. I realize leaders have challenging jobs and often are simply doing the best they can with the information they have. But we're witnessing a direction in medicine that I've never seen before in my entire career. Science is about asking questions, looking at the data, making assessments and adjustments as needed — all based on what the evidence shows. But now just raising questions or challenging the accepted narrative has put my medical license at risk. That's tough on me, I won't deny it."

"I know," she responded. "I heard, and I feel bad for you."

Nancy grew quiet as she sensed my own exasperation, and true to her nature, in spite of her anguish, she tried to encourage me: "Dr. Jensen, I appreciate your speaking out and what you post on social media. I was proud of you for challenging the directives to more casually classify deaths as being COVID-related!"

She went on, "My nurse friend who works in St. Paul has told me a lot about what is going on. She's absolutely bothered by what she is seeing in her hospital, but she's afraid that if she speaks up she could lose her job. She thinks people are dying who could be saved. She says that many doctors she works with every day are struggling with how to best care for their patients. But she won't say anything publicly. Honestly, Dr. Jensen, I don't recognize my country anymore. I'm scared."

Seeing Nancy's anxiety — born of the never-ending media fear-mongering — made me angry. And then came the plea that I have heard a thousand times. Desperate for some morsel of hope, she asked, "How do we get back to normal?"

"Nancy," I responded, "to be honest, I don't know what 'normal' is anymore, let alone how to get back there. The whole world's gone a bit crazy. Lockdowns have been used for nearly two years — needlessly, I now think. We've been told both to wear masks and then NOT to wear masks. We've been forced to isolate older family members, and then watched these vulnerable loved ones die alone. Why? This isn't Ebola. We shut down the world and seem to be on our way to bankrupting it — all for a virus that has a 99.997% recovery rate for most healthy folks under 50. I'm sorry, Nancy. I don't know how we get back to normal."

Not what she was hoping to hear, Nancy's frustration bubbled over. "Dr. Jensen, now the government has put on a full-court press to vaccinate everyone. Why? A shot that doesn't prevent infection or stop the spread is touted as a miracle cure. I don't get it. This is not how medicine should be practiced!"

She wasn't finished. "Something's terribly wrong, Dr. Jensen. I know it. I just don't know who's doing what. I don't know who to blame. Is it government? Is there a plan? Is it about power and *control? I don't know. But something is just not right."*

Somewhat lamely I answered, "Nancy, I hear you. I don't know what to say."

With that our discussion was over, and after I addressed her complaint about a tender ankle, Nancy left the clinic, subdued and unsatisfied.

* * *

My conversation with Nancy raised some important issues for which I did not have ready answers — or perhaps more accurately, answers I was very reluctant to offer. Truthfully, her questions, combined with my own experience and research, were leading me in a direction I did not want to go.

I pride myself in being an honest, albeit skeptical, person. In my world, feelings often play second fiddle to facts, even if such a prioritization might be hurtful to some. If things don't seem right, don't add up, or don't make sense, my normal *modus operandi* is to ask questions and challenge any assumptions. I can't help myself. It is a true obsession.

But the discussion with Nancy put me on a path of self-examination I was reluctant to travel. Her relentless quest for answers I couldn't provide created a sense of guilt, because I recognized that I had somehow convinced myself that it was okay for me not to come to grips with such questions. My conversation with Nancy sparked a realization that I needed to aggressively pursue the truth behind the questions she had raised — and I had been avoiding. Was my reluctance somehow connected to anxiety over the truth I might be forced to face? Was there a fear that the answers to those questions might open a door I did not want to go through — perhaps a door of no return?

Nancy had, indeed, created a conundrum for me. Why had I been willing to let lingering and unsatisfied questions go unexplored? Why had I so casually allowed my mind to take a pass on issues I knew were important and unresolved?

In this stream of thought I recognized that I had preferred to remain in the comfortable space of concluding, "We don't know enough yet." I had chosen to accept a place of safe ignorance rather than confronting what might prove to be an inconvenient and unpleasant truth — a truth that would be irrevocably disruptive.

My courage had failed me. Remaining in the comfort zone of accepting the conventional media that sounded plausible, and even somewhat reasonable, had kept me from digging deeper for the real truth.

I had been blinded by my own normalcy bias. Nancy had pushed me to confront my comfortable assumption that the answers to my questions were not presently available. I had allowed my strong sense of what I typically considered to be "normal" to serve as an acceptable rationale for not demanding answers to questions I knew deep inside needed to be asked.

A willingness to let my internal bias determine what normal looked like held me back from pursuing the answers I could have pursued — and should have pursued. My internal desire to maintain a sense of "normal" compelled me to decide that avoiding my own unresolved questions was preferable to a hard-nosed search which might reveal that my presumption of what was "normal" was terribly misplaced.

Unwittingly, that normalcy bias had become the preferred lens through which I viewed the COVID world, and which allowed my unsettled concerns to go unchallenged for the sake of "peace of mind." Sadly, I allowed myself to embrace the dishonest conclusion that some questions and queries had no clear answers — or, perhaps, were better left buried.

You see, I would not normally believe that there are evil people with nefarious plans who are actually willing to harm thousands of people, whether it be for money or power. And yet, the sad truth is that such people do, indeed, exist. Most of us are decent, hardworking and honest folk, and my life experiences have convinced me that people care for one another in times of crisis and difficulty. That is the way I look at the world and that is the general opinion I hold of others.

While I'm not so naïve as to realize there are some bad people among us, for me that's certainly not "the norm." And therein lies the seedbed of my "normalcy bias." Because I don't think like a homicidal megalomaniac, I presume that no one else could either. Yet the entirety of history boldly contradicts that presumption. There has always been an exclusive group of individuals willing and ready to use power in ways that would be abhorrent to the vast majority of humanity. And by allowing my normalcy bias to blind me to that reality, I had unwittingly hidden myself in a cocoon of dangerous ignorance.

I had to pause and reflect on this for a long moment. I clearly remembered Nancy declaring with conviction: *"Something's terribly wrong, Dr. Jensen. I know it. I just don't know who's doing what. I don't know who to blame. Is it government? Is there a plan?*

Is it about power and control? I don't know. But something is just not right."

Likewise, I clearly recalled my response to her concern: I had declared uncertainty, shut down the discussion, and attended to her sore ankle.

How should I have responded? Perhaps something like the following:

Nancy, I wish I could say something that would make all this easier, but I am having the same struggle as you. I don't want to blame anybody, because I can't find it within myself to imagine that someone could willingly orchestrate the things that have happened during this COVID crisis. I believe, by and large, that people are good, and that it would be impossible, unthinkable for people — people we have trusted and assumed had our best interest in mind — to do terrible and evil things. In the same manner I have a hard time accepting the notion that everyday bureaucrats and politicians would willingly slant the truth to advance barbaric agendas. And yet, I fully realize that Big Government could use emergency powers to inflate Big Pharma revenues, and this collusion could easily be hidden from the public eye by Big Tech companies cancelling noisy and distracting contrarian voices.

However, I must confess that I am finding it more and more difficult to hold to my typical mindset that nefarious behaviors are not likely. Rather I am finding it more and more credible that ultimately we will learn that people and companies were willing to deceive and cheat the general citizenry.

I still don't know what the truth is. But I do know that if we're going to learn what we need to learn so that a pandemic like this and the policies surrounding it never happen again, then we have to correctly diagnose the real situation, and determine what is true, what is not, and what we are really facing — regardless of our own internal biases. If my bias toward an assumed normalcy blinds me to the truth, then I won't be a part of any solution going forward; I will be part of the problem that keeps all of us in the dark.

But I did not say any of this to Nancy. Instead, I had needed time, time to think, time to get smarter — time to challenge myself to be ruthlessly honest with what was happening all around me. Only then could I find a way to break through my normalcy bias so I could discover the truth to a crisis that had become the transformational event of my lifetime. And Nancy would have to discover her own truths as well.

Obstacles are put in our way to see if what we want is worth FIGHTING FOR.

—Anonymous

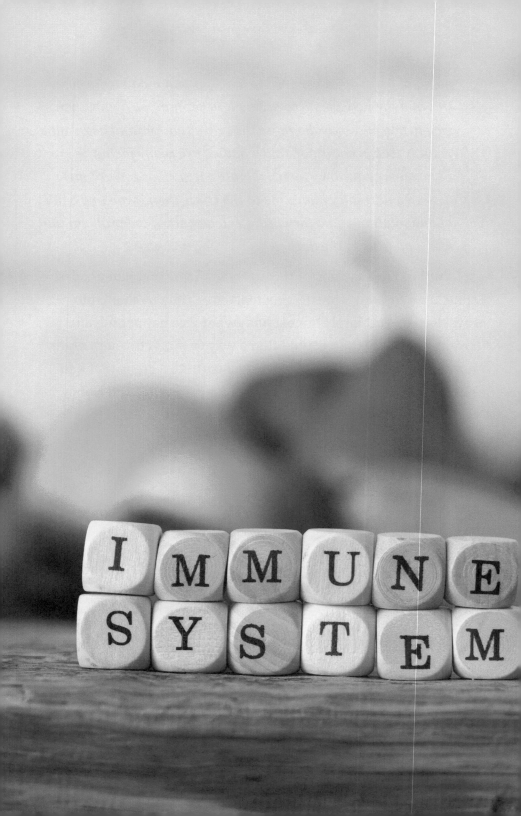

CHAPTER TWENTY THREE

BUILDING
STRONG
IMMUNITY

I frequently get letters, e-mails, and queries from patients wanting to know how to strengthen their immune systems. Following is a note I received not long ago that is typical of what people want to know:

> *Dr. Jensen, I don't want to take any of the COVID vaccines. I have investigated multiple resources, including the CDC's VAERS [Vaccine Adverse Event Reporting System] data bank, and I am concerned that serious side effects have been documented in thousands of people who have taken any one of these vaccines. What are some everyday actions you recommend that might strengthen my immune system and perhaps help me against COVID if I do get it? — Your patient, Megan.*

To Megan and the countless other individuals who are seeking practical advice on how to maintain a healthy lifestyle in our present COVID-impacted world, my typical recommendations are as follows:

- Strive for a healthy lifestyle that incorporates good nutrition, fresh air, sunlight (within reason), and exercises that strengthen and stretch your muscles as well as exercises that give your cardiovascular system a workout.

- Maintain a reasonable body weight (BMI less than 30).

- Don't smoke or use recreational drugs, and let moderation be your guide with alcohol consumption.

- Learn how to de-stress by practicing daily meditation. Seek the best rest at night you can get.

- In addition to the above lifestyle opportunities, I also recommend that you consider some of the following nutritional supplements in moderation to keep your immune system functioning at its best:

Vitamin C is a water-soluble nutrient well known for its vital role in maintaining a healthy immune system. It has been shown to help prevent or mitigate against viral, bacterial, and other infections by acting as a natural antihistamine and anti-inflammatory agent. Vitamin C is necessary for the production of collagen (a structural protein in connective tissue), and is therefore important for skin, bone, and joint health. Vitamin C is needed for amino acid metabolism, neuro-transmitter synthesis, and the utilization of many other nutrients such as folic acid and iron. It is also an effective antioxidant that can help maintain healthy tissues by neutralizing free radicals generated during normal metabolism and exposure to environmental stressors.

Vitamin D is an important immune system-strengthening nutrient that can reduce the risk of colds and flu. It is fat-soluable and can be stored in the body. Exposure to natural sunlight is a critical source of vitamin D during the summer months. Unfortunately, from late September through mid-May in the Northern Hemisphere it is challenging to get adequate vitamin D from sunlight alone. Some physicians contend that low vitamin D levels are the rule rather than the exception in Northern Hemispheric winters. You should consider supplementation with vitamin D during the late autumn and winter months when exposure to natural sunlight is limited.

Vitamin E is a fat-soluble vitamin that can act as an antioxidant and eliminate free radicals that can damage cells. It also enhances immune function and may slow the process of hardening of the arteries. Antioxidant vitamins, including vitamin E, came to public attention in the 1980s when scientists began to understand that free-radical damage was involved in the early stages of artery-clogging atherosclerosis, and might also contribute to cancer, vision loss, and a host of other chronic conditions. Vitamin E has the ability to protect cells from free-radical damage, as well as reduce the production of free radicals in certain situations.

Vitamin A, when used on a short-term basis, can help support the body's ability to fight infections, especially respiratory infections.

Zinc can help reduce the number of infections and the duration of the common cold when taken within 24 hours of onset. It impedes viral replication.

Selenium is a key nutrient for immune function and is easily obtained from foods like the Brazil nut. Selenium is also an antioxidant which strengthens the body's defenses against bacteria, viruses, and cancer cells.

Garlic in fresh, aged extract, and supplement forms may reduce the severity of upper viral respiratory infections such as the common cold.

Probiotics contain "good bacteria" that both support gut health and influence the function and regulation of the immune system. They can also decrease the number of respiratory infections, especially in children.

Quercetin is a type of flavonoid antioxidant found in plant foods, including leafy greens, tomatoes, berries, and broccoli. Quercetin is considered one of the most abundant antioxidants in the human diet, and plays an important part in fighting free-radical damage. It also assists the entry of zinc into cells, which is likely very important in corona virus infections.

Elderberry appears to have properties that may help to fight viruses, according to recent studies.

It is important to understand that these supplements are suggestions, and more research needs to be done to fully understand the additional benefits they may offer. Just like exercise, I personally recommend taking the most reasonable beneficial dose possible when supplementing with vitamins and minerals. I don't recommend mega-dosing on any of these supplements, because if you overdo it, you can overtax your vital organs and rather than being a tremendous benefit, these efforts can become a detriment.

Most of my recommendations are low-cost and center on the notion that you are your own best champion when it comes to your health. I would also note that there is not always a lot of good research around these suggestions because Big Pharma is not likely to generate big profits from everyday over-the-counter supplements and may be disinclined to fund research on them.

My personal recommendation for all individuals is that you work with your healthcare team to help determine the most beneficial supplements and dosages for you.

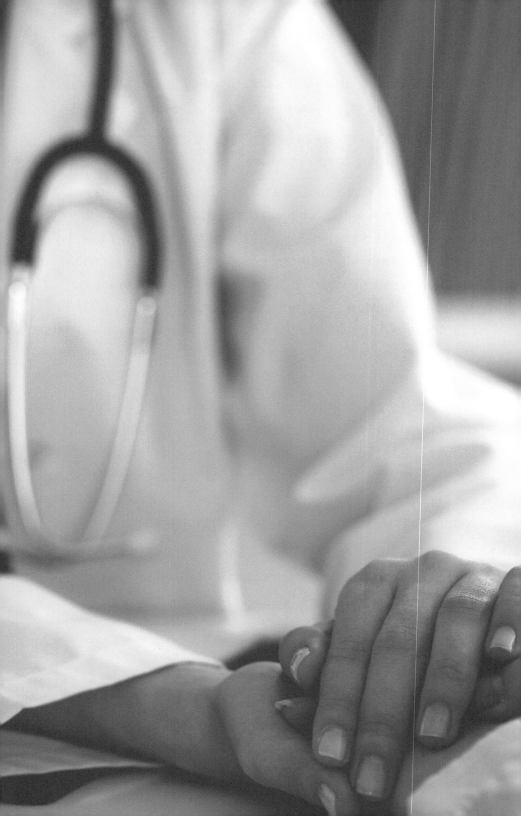

CHAPTER TWENTY FOUR

The Miracle of
CARING

I had just finished seeing a patient when my nurse told me I had a call waiting for me.

"Hi, Dr. Scott Jensen here. How can I help you?"

The voice on the other end was that of Julie, a long-ago patient who saw me as a teenager when she sprained her ankle at a high school sporting event. It was hard to believe that thirty years had passed.

"Dr. Jensen, it's my dad. He's very weak, and he's been sick for five days. I think he's got COVID, but he won't let me take him to the emergency room. He even told me, 'Julie, if you take me there, I'll never come home again.' I didn't know what to do. You're his doctor and about the only person he'll listen to. I'm sorry to bother you, but I just don't know where to turn."

As I listened to Julie, I thought of how many times I had heard similar stories since COVID turned the world upside down in 2020.

"Where's Henry now?" I asked.

"He's here with us. We brought him to our house and set up a bed in the family room."

"Good, having him close by keeps him reassured and makes it easier to watch him."

I asked a few more questions and then said, "Julie, why don't you give me your address and I'll stop over around six when I'm done here at the clinic? I can get a better feel for how your dad is doing if I can listen to his lungs and check him over."

She sounded surprised. "Dr. Jensen, you mean you'll make a house call?"

"Sure, it's easier for me to come to Henry than for him to come

to me. It sounds like it would be tough for you to load him into your car. And it's icy out. Does six work for you?"

I could hear the relief in Julie's voice, "That would be great. Thanks so much. Oh, and by the way — my husband was able to get some ivermectin. Do you think I can start giving that to Dad?"

"Julie, let's wait on that for now," I responded. "I'll review his chart and see him in a couple of hours, and we can talk it over then."

Two hours later I was greeting Henry face-to-face. Walking into his makeshift bedroom told me a lot. I marveled at how a home could be reshaped in the wake of a serious illness. Here was a family room fitted out with an adjustable bed, commode, bedpan, serving trays, and folding chairs. All this surrounded a tough-looking guy who obviously hadn't shaved or showered in a few days. Henry was a vigorous 75-year-old man who now had shadows under his eyes, hollowed-out cheeks, and pasty-looking skin that matched the color of his white bedsheets. He had aged a lot since I had last seen him.

"Hi, Henry," I said as I approached his bed.

He swiveled his head, nodded at me, and a smile appeared. "Thanks for coming, Doc. I didn't think you made house calls anymore."

I chuckled, "I do what I must when I'm trying to keep a stubborn old man from driving his family nuts! Julie told me that the hospital is out of the question. Is that right?"

"For sure, that's right, Doc. I've heard stories down at the Legion about folks going in and can't get out, unless they're taking a taxi ride in a hearse. So, no, I'm not going to any hospital. And I'll be darned if I'm going to have some of those rip-off drugs that cost *an arm and a leg injected into my body!"*

"Fair enough, Henry. Your body, your choice. So let's take a look at you. It's nice to see you again. How long has it been now?"

And we were off to the races. He wasn't doing great. His breathing was rapid and shallow, his pulse was high, blood pressure low. But his oxygen levels were okay, no fever, and his tongue was moist. He wasn't in any distress. After further scrutiny, I cleared my throat and shared my thoughts.

"Henry, Julie, let's go ahead and presume we're dealing with COVID."

I talked and they listened. Then they talked and I listened. Together we put together a plan. Medicines were reviewed, side effects were discussed, and I advised them as to what to watch for regarding worsening conditions.

I understood where he was coming from, and I certainly couldn't blame him for not wanting to go to the hospital. In the wake of the COVID-19 pandemic and the way it had been portrayed in the media, was it any wonder that men like Henry were beyond fearful? His attitude of angry skepticism could not be changed. The truth was that Henry was convinced that a hospitalization would end in death.

But Henry did well. I stayed close and in-touch. I rechecked his lungs when he came to the clinic three weeks later. His words were few.

"Thanks, Doc. You saved my life. I won't forget it."

His smile was broad and his handshake was firm. He left without another word, and I said a prayer of thanks.

* * *

There were other reasons I made a house call to check on Henry. He wasn't willing to go to the hospital, but at the same time I didn't want him coming to my clinic. Exposing employees and patients was something our entire staff tried to avoid. We had masks and protective personal equipment and took a host of protective measures to avoid possible transmission.

We did not want to spread this disease. I personally had recovered from COVID and had donated plasma to help others who were struggling. My array of antibodies was something the blood bank people boasted about and couldn't get enough of. So a house call was a measure I was willing to take.

A Final Takeaway

The COVID-19 pandemic did many things to families, communities, and society as a whole. One of the worst things that happened was the fracturing of the relationship between patients and their healthcare team.

It's time we reclaim an essential ingredient that has been disappearing from the medical profession: a deep commitment to real connections between patients and healers — because only then can we rediscover the miracle of really caring for others.

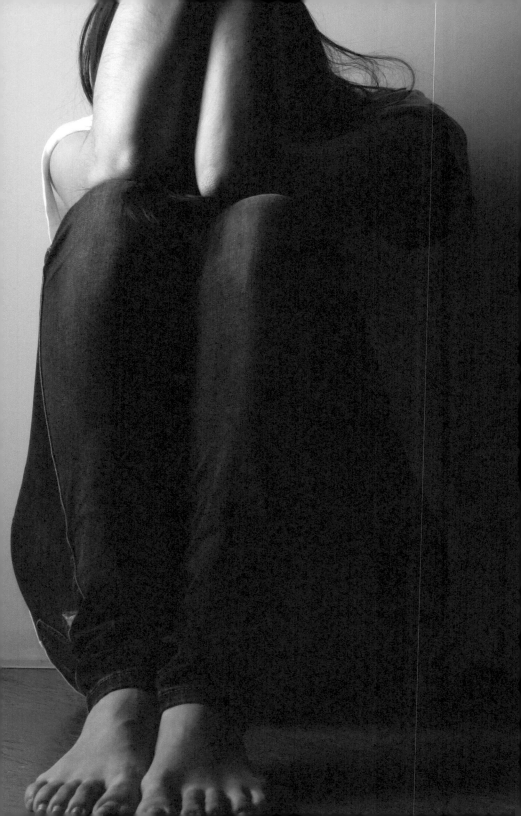

CHAPTER TWENTY FIVE

SOUND THE ALARM— KIDS ARE DYING

I stepped into the exam room and there sat Will, a patient of mine since he was a three-year-old toddler. Now, 18 years later, Will was a handsome young man with a long list of academic and athletic achievements. I was proud to be his doctor and had long enjoyed his bright and cheerful personality.

But today he was not his usual self. In fact, Will was glum. I'd never seen him like this.

"Hi, Will, how're you doing?"

He shrugged, "Okay, I guess."

"How was your holiday break?" I ventured. "Did you do anything fun?"

This time Will looked me straight in the eye and said tersely: "How exactly would I do that, Dr. Jensen? I couldn't take my girlfriend out on a date with all the stupid restrictions. My friends all hunkered down in their basements playing video games, and since I don't play, I'm pretty much out of their loop. My parents told me to quit moping around, but all they do is watch the news and bicker."

The long silence that followed spoke volumes.

"Will, how can I help?"

He stared at his shoes and stammered a bit without looking at me. "I guess I'm here because me and a couple of friends got vaccinated a few months ago so we could play sports at the university. A week later one of them was diagnosed with a heart issue, and I wonder if I should be worried."

His voice and body language told me there was more to his visit than that.

"I'm glad you're here, Will," I answered. "We'll check out your heart and lungs. No problem doing that right now."

After reviewing his history and doing an exam and electrocardiogram, I told Will that there was no issue with his heart. That brought a nod and Will hesitantly stood, apparently to leave.

"Thanks, Dr. Jensen, I appreciate your help."

"Will," I said, "something else is going on, isn't there? I've got some time. I just had a couple of cancellations, so I'm in no rush. What else should we be talking about?"

With that Will broke down and the tears flowed. We sat there together and the room was quiet — a long time. Then Will choked out words I'll never forget.

"I'm sorry. I haven't been straight up."

I waited.

"My buddies are dead," he began. "They both committed suicide. The one with the heart issue had been doing okay, and we all talked about getting back to school and living a normal college life. But that didn't happen. Life on campus didn't get any better. It was worse, and the rules kept coming. 'Do this, don't do that.' Every week things got darker. We weren't really living. We were just going through the motions. Nothing got better, and then one night I guess something snapped for Billy. He killed himself. And a month later Karl did the same. I couldn't believe it — I still can't."

Silence.

"And now — now I catch myself wondering, wondering if that's a path I'll take."

I could barely speak. "I'm sorry, Will, so sorry."

He continued: "I've been doing a lot of thinking and wondering — what's the use? Does anything really matter?"

I said nothing.

He sobbed a bit and his shoulders shook. I put my hand on the back of his and sat — and waited.

After a while I asked, "Will, can I call your folks?"

Finally, a nod.

Will's parents showed up and together the four of us put a plan together.

Over the subsequent weeks and months Will did okay. But we all realized we were not out of the woods. Will needed time. And Will needed normalcy. And for a lifetime, Will needed healing.

* * *

On October 17, 2019, four months before the COVID pandemic was officially declared in 2020, the National Center for Health Statistics (NCHS) released *Data Brief #352*. The headline read: "Death Rates Due to Suicide and Homicide Among Persons Aged 10-24: United States, 2000-2017."

I had been intrigued to dig into the article to discover what the statistics had to say about the state of mental health among America's younger generation. Since my own brother's suicide many years ago, I had always puzzled about the moment someone actually made the commitment to end his or her life — the only earthly one they would get.

The report had a profound impact on me. In essence the data from the NCHS revealed that during the decade from 2007 to

2017, suicide had increased by an incredible 56 percent among young people in the 10- to 24-year-old age group. It stated that after stable trends from 2000 to 2007, suicide rates for persons aged 10–24 increased from 6.8 per 100,000 persons in 2007, to 10.6 persons per 100,000 in 2017.

Mental health experts had been sounding the alarm about a catastrophic wave of youth suicide well before the COVID pandemic. In fact, suicide was officially the second leading cause of death for older teens and young adults with one in four admitting that they had suicidal thoughts on a frequent basis.

And the situation was likely worse than the data represented. Dr. Victor M. Fornari, the vice chair of child and adolescent psychiatry at Zucker Hillside Hospital in Glen Oaks, New York, was quoted as saying: "Even though the study by the CDC demonstrates an increased rate of completed suicide in the adolescent, young adult age group, I still think we need to recognize that suicide may be underreported, and that accidents continue to be the leading cause of death and a significant number of those accidents may actually have been suicide."

I understood that multiple biological, psychological, and social factors came into play, making it difficult to pinpoint one sole reason for the surge in teen suicide. Numerous common risk factors, including hormonal imbalances, anxiety, depression, trauma, family history, and alcohol/drug use contributed greatly to this societal catastrophe.

But something was clearly changing. I suspected that cell phones, social media bullying, and newly born pressures were exerting harmful and immeasurable influences on the lives of young people.

And to add fuel to the fire, the devastating impacts of unpredictable COVID-19 curfews, closures, lockdowns, and other rigid restrictions, along with haphazard enforcement created combustible circumstances in all sorts of places.

Disrupted relationships in social, work, and family settings combined with the added uncertainty of not knowing how long COVID conditions might last, caused many young people to suffer from a gnawing sense that their best years were being stolen from them. Their lives, freedom, and opportunities were being suffocated.

Around the world younger generations lost economic opportunities, missed traditional milestone events, and forfeited human connections. Many felt they were being forced to pay a huge personal price — not because of the pandemic's risk to them personally, but because of the draconian measures supposedly necessary to protect the vulnerable. A fractured society was demanding impossible and involuntary sacrifices.

The despair faced by younger generations was transformational in a way that easily coaxed thoughts of suicide from even the most secure of mindsets.

The long-lasting duration of the COVID-19 pandemic unveiled the folly of so many government interventions, many of which seemed to represent unnecessary, inconsistent, and ineffective intrusions on individual liberties. This almost casual willingness to inflict such relentless assaults on human freedom will be a lasting element of the COVID pandemic's legacy.

While Big Government policies cultivated suicidal thoughts and actions in too many young people, this path of spiritual destruction was obviously greased by the insidious impact of Big Tech on our culture, particularly that of younger generations. The irresistible "drug" of social media platforms like Facebook and Instagram — with the relentless pursuit of likes, shares, comments, and engagements — too often led to emotions of depression, despair, and anxiety as young people starving for acceptance and belonging found themselves "unfriended," cancelled, ignored, or shunned for a variety of reasons, or for no reason at all.

And so it was that in 2019 the CDC sounded the alarm: kids are dying. This proclamation of a rising wave of youth suicide did not foretell the tsunami of suicides yet to come.

My clinic experiences over the last couple of years have indeed revealed a distressing increase of feelings of foreboding, confusion, and despair among young adults. Too often such attitudes overtake the mind and lead to a decision by a young person that ending his or her life is the only viable option.

And while Big Pharma may claim to have the remedies for chemical imbalances, anxiety, depression, trauma, family history, alcohol, and drugs, in the matter of mental illness, I am long past buying what the drug companies are selling. Their oversimplification for addressing problems of the mind and soul has too often been gross and unhelpful in the matter of restoring the joy of living.

We must find a path not yet discovered.

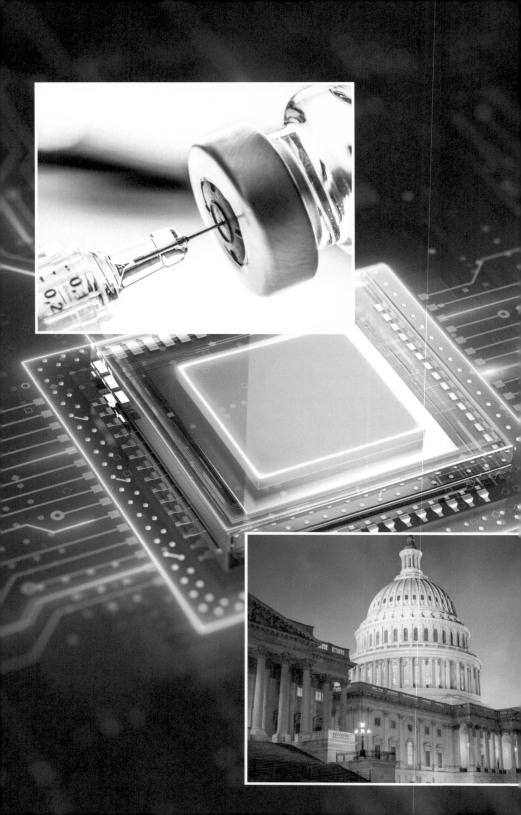

CHAPTER TWENTY SIX

TRIAD of POWER-BROKERS

"Facts are stubborn things; and whatever may be our wishes, our inclinations, or the dictates of our passion, they cannot alter the state of facts and evidence."

— John Adams

FOUNDING FATHER, SECOND PRESIDENT OF THE UNITED STATES

In my 2015 book *Relationship Matters*, I wrote:

The foundation of medical care is the time-honored connection between patient and doctor, and it relies on trust and advocacy. Unfortunately, it is fracturing and has been fracturing for some time.

Skyrocketing insurance premiums providing less coverage, big business maneuverings, expanding government intrusion, entitlement programs running short of funds, increasing costs associated with dying, and risky interventions threatening the patient — all these elements serve to create a combustible medical milieu with the fuse already lit.

Navigating the twenty-first century healthcare maze is no easy task — for patients or physicians — and already many personal choices have been taken out of patients' hands. A paradigm shift is occurring in the provision and reception of healthcare services — the crisis is real, and the stakes are high. Lives will be changed. What is the end game? Who will decide what services a patient receives and when and by whom? Who will lead the quest for a solution? These are tough questions in search of elusive answers with only one thing for certain: <u>the survival of patient-driven, physician-guided healthcare is at risk.</u>

Even back in 2015 when I wrote those words, a push toward authoritarian control over America's citizens via the convergence of Big Pharma, Big Tech, and Big Government — which I now refer to as the Triad of Tyranny — was already evident.

The issue I addressed back then is the same issue I address now, only with far greater immediacy and with clear evidence made manifest to each and every American since the COVID-19 pandemic began in early 2020. Each of us has experienced a dramatic loss of our constitutionally guaranteed freedoms as government forces have imposed lockdowns, shutdowns, lock-ins, lock-outs, mandates, distancing, masking, and vaccinations — while concurrently and arbitrarily suppressing or restricting access to medical evaluations, treatments, and interventions which could have saved lives.

This autocratic level of control and restriction could only have been accomplished by the convergence of Big Pharma, Big Tech, and Big Government, a Triad of Tyranny, colluding together. Think about it. We have all seen and experienced firsthand the restrictions and mandatory controls imposed on our nation's economy and its people. It is a real crisis we all face, in a real way. No one is exempt.

Simply put, there is only one way out of the present healthcare crisis, and the dilemma we face centers on the need for patients and doctors to work together to reclaim our system of healers healing those in need. Patients must force the dismantling of this Triad of Tyranny and restore balance, advocacy, and trust to the matter of giving and receiving healthcare.

My goal is to galvanize both patients and doctors to commit to rebuilding the vital relationships they once enjoyed — bonds that can make the difference between good or bad care, relief or suffering, even life or death.

Let me offer a real-life example that happened not long ago when I met with two of my long-term patients, Tilly and George.

* * *

It was a familiar scene I had seen played out many times before as I walked into the exam room. There was George sitting and scowling as Tilly fussed with her hearing aids. I'm not sure why, but on that day I sensed our visit was going to be a bit tense.

Tilly had chronically nagged George about various things and didn't seem to know when to quit. When she volunteered information about his bad diet or too many beers, he mocked her. And yet, most of the information she provided was reliable.

George, on the other hand, fibbed uncontrollably; if allowed to, he could finish a case of beer in a weekend and tell me it had lasted a month! He might scoff at Tilly's recollections, but beyond his bluster, he knew how much Tilly loved him and that her story was closer to reality than his. In fact, once in a great while, when I least expected it, I'd catch him with a slight smile and nodding his head in appreciation regarding some comment she had added. Sometimes I smiled to myself as I listened to their back-and-forth banter, and I wondered how they had weathered more than forty years together.

As I sat down, I commented to Tilly, "That's a pretty sweater, Tilly."

She beamed.

"Hey, George, how're you doing today?"

A grunt was followed by a burp. Tilly — embarrassed — looked down and stared at her feet as I waited.

Without any provocation, George launched into a tirade, "Darn it, Doc, the TV ads made it sound like once-a-week shots would almost cure my diabetes. Last time I was in, you told me my numbers looked great, and you and I were both happy campers. But I gotta tell you, as much as I'd like to, I just can't afford to continue these weekly injections. At first the drug company's coupon program worked out okay and made it possible for me to try it. But now things have changed, and it's costing me $300 every month out of pocket. That's way beyond what I can handle. So, I tried going to an injection every three weeks, but now my sugars have gone way up."

As I listened carefully and glanced at his chart, I readily understood why his A1C lab test had skyrocketed so far out of the desirable range. When George felt he could no longer maintain the recommended weekly interval for his injections, and instead tried to stretch the interval, his sugars went wild.

George continued, "It kind of ticks me off, Doc. At the start I told you I didn't think I could afford the newfangled drugs. But you were good about helping me get on the manufacturer's assistance program, so I went along with it. Now my wife's chewing me out every day because my sugar numbers aren't as good as they were. It sort of feels like a bait-and-switch job. They baited me into using their meds with their glitzy TV ads and promises. And now that I've gotten used to the medicine and good numbers, they pull the rug out from under me and want to charge me three times as much. I'm sorry, Doc, I don't have the money to do what you want me to do. It's as simple as that. Now my sugars suck. I get that and I'm not making any excuses. But I do feel like I got played, and I'm not happy."

Tilly chimed in, "Well, maybe if you cut down on the beer and the chips, you'd be doing better."

I shook my head and interrupted before Tilly could say anything more. "George, I know you're trying. Let's forget about what we can't do and step back and take a look at what we can do. We'll make this work somehow. We've got some options."

Tilly jumped in. "Dr. Jensen, there's more you need to know. It isn't just the cost of George's medicines that's making his diabetes a real problem. His workplace has been really tough on him. George and the other workers often get caught up in what they post on social media, and their boss doesn't stop it. Some of the employees have posted nasty comments about George taking too many breaks because he can't control his sugar numbers. Others gang up on him and tease him that no one else with the same insurance coverage is having any problems paying for their medicines. I swear, the Internet and Facebook make it sound like only idiots have a hard time taking care of their diabetes, and that's not fair because I know how hard George has tried. I don't like the bullying that goes on in social media, but how do you stop it? An awful lot of people have no idea how hard it can be to handle diabetes when you first get diagnosed in your sixties, and the Internet isn't helping one bit!"

I thought Tilly was done, but she continued.

"When George gets mad, he gets stupid, and he has posted some pretty mean insults back at his fellow workers. Now they think he's a jerk, and they're mad. They complained to Facebook and his boss. Facebook put him in jail for a week. I'm not sure what his boss

might do. I worry that he's going to get fired.

George cut in. "Come on, Tilly, I'm not getting fired because of social media. I've been at the plant for more than 25 years and they need me. But you're right. I didn't do myself any favors with what I posted. I was just fed up with all the crap."

George turned to me, and in a voice touched with emotion he said, "Doc, it's been a tough few weeks, and Tilly, please don't bother saying anything more. I hear you."

I let the emotions in the room cool down.

George had more to say. "You wanna know what else is going on now? The company is making us tell them whether or not we got vaccinated because President Biden said all companies with more than 100 workers had to mandate the vaccine. Whatever happened to health privacy? Doc, you treated me and I was out for a week with COVID last year, so my boss knows I already had it. You checked my antibodies and told me they were good. So what the heck is going on? How can the government force me to tell my employer about my health history? And how can they demand that I get a vaccine to get antibodies I already got? Where are my rights?"

It was my turn. "George, I understand what you're saying. It's an odd world we live in these days."

Tilly interrupted. "You know what else, Dr. Jensen? Another thing that makes me angry is this stuff about 'informed consent.' You know how you or your nurse always asks us to sign that form before you do anything to us. You tell us what's up and how you're gonna do such and such, and then we sign a form that says we've provided informed consent. Well, George isn't getting informed and he sure as heck isn't consenting. Instead he gets bullied, and now they're trying to force him into taking a vaccine he doesn't want. Down the road I could see it getting bad enough that if he won't take the vaccine, he could get fired. Government shouldn't be able to do that to us."

I could not have agreed more.

George chimed in, "Doc, the world's crazy! I just don't get what's going on. A few weeks ago one of my buddies at work got COVID and went to the hospital. His cousin had gotten over COVID just a couple months earlier with some kind of medicine that used to be easy to get, but when my buddy asked for it, they told him he couldn't have it. The doctor said the government wasn't allowing that medicine to be used. What happened to a patient's 'right to try'?"

"I hear you both loud and clear," I responded. "I don't have the answers, and I sure didn't make the rules. George, I appreciate hearing what's going on in your life, but let's press pause on our discussion of current affairs and take a look at you."

A little while later, the exam was over, and I had revised George's medication plan to eliminate the expensive injections and add a couple of generic pills. They left, mollified but still on edge.

* * *

Back in my office I thought about how citizens in our country represent less than five percent of the world's population, and yet they take nearly 40 percent of the world's prescriptions and more than 80 percent of its opioids. I thought about the impact Big Pharma wields on the American economy and on our everyday lives. The truth is the pharmaceutical industry, as a major component of the Triad of Tyranny, has gotten to the point that it can control doctors, patients, research centers, universities, politicians, and many more stakeholders. When and how does this domination get stopped?

I found myself wondering how it had gotten to the point that I had to warn patients to be cautious about what they shared with doctors or revealed to hospital workers, because whatever they say might end up in their chart, and it may not be conducive to a good outcome. How was I to let my patients know that their government is constantly collecting their personal data?

As I pondered these issues I realized that my mood had soured. I resented that anything I said — anything at all — could find its way onto social media, be distorted, and could then prompt complaints against me. Social media platforms had become very aggressive about shutting people down if something showed up on their page that wasn't consistent with the narrative the given platform had approved. I couldn't help but wonder how we had gotten into this mess.

* * *

There was a knock at my office door, and there stood George. He hemmed and hawed a bit and finally stammered, "I just want to apologize, Doc, for not being straight up with you about not taking the injections the way you wanted me to. I know you work hard to help me with my diabetes, and I feel like I let you down."

I shook my head and said, "George, we're in this thing together. I know you're trying. I want to do everything in my power to help you be your own best champion for your health. Only you know what you can afford and I appreciate you shooting straight with me about it. I'm here to help you be as healthy as you can be. Let's work together. You can count on me to go to bat for you, and I

*know you trust me. We both feel like we've been played — Big
Pharma with its tempting coupon programs, Big Government with
its data collection, and Big Tech with its willingness to cancel you
if it chooses, and never mind its willingness to distort and massage
the truth. It's a tough world we live in right now, and so much feels
so ugly! But my job is to help you be the champion of your health.
No one can do it as well as you. And I'll do everything I can to help."*

*George nodded, grunted, and slapped me on the shoulder,
"Thanks, Doc, you're all right."*

*He walked away, and as I slowly closed the door I detected
a lump in my throat. George had gotten to me emotionally. He
touched me with his simple and sincere apology for not being an
ideal patient.*

* * *

I sat at my desk a long time considering that powerbrokers
like Big Pharma, Big Tech, and Big Government would never
voluntarily recalibrate what they do or how they do it. I
understood that left unchecked and unchallenged, it wasn't even
possible for this tyrannical triad to focus on the common good
of the American people — not as long as its stakeholders were
shackled to the almighty dollar and ever-expanding power.

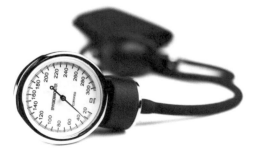

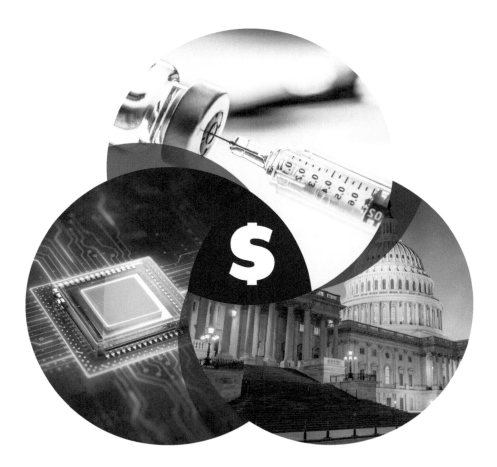

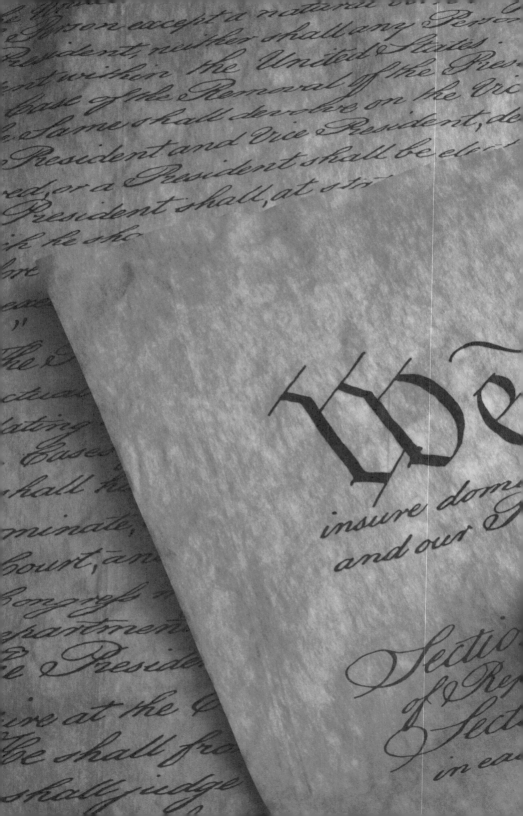

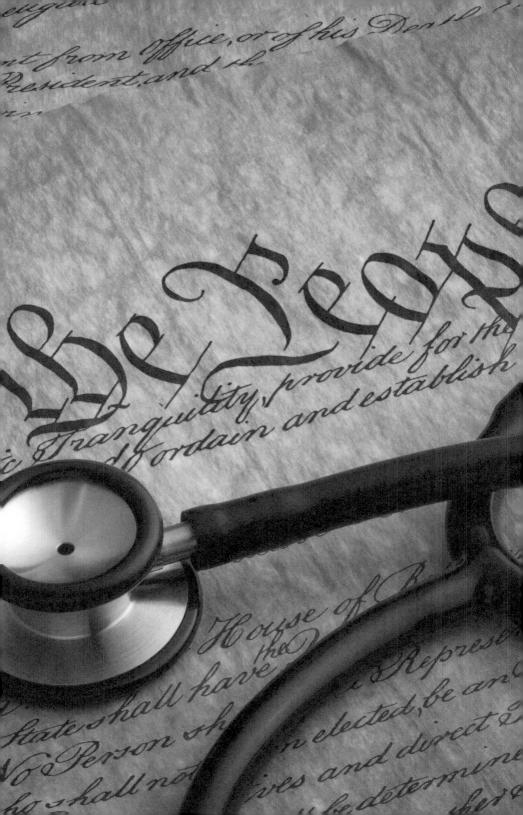

AFTERWORD

"If the soul is left in darkness, sins will be committed.
The guilty one is not he who commits the sin,
but the one who causes the darkness."
— Victor Hugo, *Les Misérables*

The America in which I grew up during the last half of the 20th century was a beacon of light and hope expressing lasting freedom throughout the world. Nevertheless, each decade was marked by contentious social, political, and health issues that sparked heated debates in all sectors of our society. However, without fail, the right to question authorities, voice opposition, and express dissent peacefully were protected by our Constitution. Mainstream media, with its newspapers, magazines, radio, and television programs, were steadfast forces in safeguarding the opportunity for the public to participate in the examination and scrutiny of the issues of the day. It was a remarkable time to be alive and witness a hallmark of post-World War II life — unrelenting free speech.

Without Debate, Without Criticism, No Republic Can Survive

I was in grade school when President John F. Kennedy addressed the American Newspaper Publishers Association on April 27, 1961. In that speech he tackled the issues of free speech and freedom of the press. Here are some excerpts:

The very word "secrecy" is repugnant in a free and open society; and we are as a people inherently and historically opposed to secret societies, to secret oaths, and to secret proceedings. We decided long ago that the dangers of excessive and unwarranted concealment of pertinent facts far outweighed the dangers which are cited to justify it.

And there is very grave danger that an announced need for increased security will be seized upon by those anxious to expand its meaning to the very limits of official censorship and concealment.

Without debate, without criticism, no Administration and no country can succeed — and no republic can survive.

Under Assault: Freedom of Speech and the Right to Dissent

Times have changed dramatically since 1961, and the 21st century now bears witness to an alarming intrusion on the rights of every American citizen to dissent and exercise freedom of thought, speech, and conscience as guaranteed by the U.S. Constitution. Indeed these liberties, heretofore often taken for granted, are under assault all over the world, but especially here in America.

The COVID-19 pandemic proved to be uniquely fertile ground for Big Pharma, Big Tech, and Big Government, the "Triad of Tyranny," to play a massive role in suppressing freedom of speech and the right to dissent, especially as related to public discussions about science, policy, and law. A new terror emerged as this Triad stretched its powerful arms and put its fingers where they had never been before.

Caught by surprise and not necessarily seeing what was happening, Americans found themselves in the midst of a different kind of epidemic — a pathologic lust for power — which had infected and infiltrated a huge part of everyday community life. The right to question and the right to know became targets in the crosshairs of the Triad. Alarmingly, even the right to choose what entered one's own body was no longer secure.

Your Right to Question, Your Right to Know, Your Right to Try

Throughout this book I have used anonymous real-life patient encounters to address issues relating to our national healthcare system which I believe must be called out: your right to question, your right to know, and your right to try. These matters need to be addressed and dissected, and solutions or protections will be in order.

The transformative COVID-19 pandemic represents a planet-wide crisis, and the very nature of future human freedoms and life on earth will depend on our collective ability to identify a path which will preserve the right to life, liberty, and the pursuit of happiness.

Never before in the history of mankind have we seen such a massive global effort to censor and silence scientific debate as during the COVID-19 pandemic. It is remarkable that in 1961 President Eisenhower cautioned Americans that there might come a day in which public policy would be held captive by a scientific and technological "elite." We have seen his warning become the eerie truth and witnessed a nationwide captivity by a small minority of powerbrokers. Indeed, a tsunami of intrusive scientific and technological forces has ushered in for many of us a new and dystopian world similar to George Orwell's nightmarish realm of *1984*, in which silencing contrarians and canceling voices was acceptable.

But this imprisonment won't last. People all over the planet are waking up, standing up, and boldly entering the arena of public debate.

Each day, citizens of the U.S. and nations around the world are becoming increasingly aware that we must collectively remain vigilant and strong in our pursuit of the truth, always being open to new data and emerging science and discovery. More than ever, the right to question and the right to know are worthy of the sacrifice they require.

A renewed realization that freedom of thought, speech, and conscience must be guarded has captured the minds and hearts of millions. A recognition that public health regulations and policies unconstitutionally restricted or eliminated civil liberties in the U.S. has given rise to a new battle cry: Freedom Above All Things. The depth and determination of this conviction revealed itself when millions of worldwide demonstrators gave support to a fifty-mile-long Canadian truckers convoy. A line of ten thousand vehicles was enough to paralyze a nation, destroy political careers, and give hope to millions.

It also gave notice to the Triad of Tyranny that our world now stands awake and invigorated with a new resolve: Never Again!

Conversations about vaccinations, mandates, passports, health freedom, informed consent, and the sanctity of the U.S. Constitution have become the order of the day, and no news sources can refrain from engaging such vital topics, no matter how much the Triad of Tyranny works to control the public narrative through its various assets.

When people feel disenfranchised and believe that those in power do not care about their lives or the lives of their children, trust in government is lost, and anger and despair become the norm. The paralyzing poison of fear-mongering may successfully produce rigid control for a time, but the two-fold antidote of skepticism and exposure is a powerful remedy.

It is a remarkable proclamation to make, but I make it here: Americans have rejected the narcotizing elixir of self-doubt, zealously promoted by the Triad of Tyranny. People around the world have chosen the wine of skepticism and protest over the forced feedings of illusion and corruption promoted by governments.

I encourage you to fan the flames of your own ferociousness. Do your research and arrive at informed conclusions. Follow your conscience — free from fear, coercion, and deceit. These are challenging times, indeed, but you will rise to this occasion. Do not doubt yourself!

Should you remain passive and disengaged, your very freedom and the right to decide what is in your own best interest will be taken from you. Do not be idle or ignorant. Now is not the time to remain silent. Let your voice be heard, and lay hold of what has been entrusted to you. It is time to be your own healthcare champion.

In an age of information, where both disinformation and misinformation abound — complicated by never-ending propaganda and political agendas — it has never been more important to accurately discern what is true. But at the same time, never before has such massive censorship, suppression, and restricted access to real data been so dominating. These are difficult times. Finding credible and trustworthy sources is increasingly challenging. But it is the raw truth that will set each of us free, so pursue it with all that is within you. Remember that your own hesitation and doubt can be your worst enemies.

May God bless all of us that we might be a light, a beacon of hope, unto one another. May we never take for granted the preciousness of our lives, the value of our liberties, and the right to pursue our happiness — unalienable rights provided by our Creator.

Live nobly and without fear.

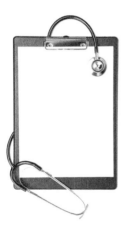

ACKNOWLEDGEMENTS

All acts of creation share similarities. There is always the need for the idea, the wondering, the research, the commitment, the starting point, the determination to finish, and finally, getting the project across the goal line.

I've formed companies, built buildings, created clinics, started restaurants, became a pilot, and written books. All of these initiatives posed difficulties, but authorship presented special challenges and demanded painstaking perseverance. Without the support of key individuals, quite frankly, this book would have no birthday.

I am incredibly indebted to the following people for their help, support, and encouragement — their combined efforts made this book a reality.

My wife, Mary, injected vital encouragement, brainstorming, and exhortation for more than two years!

My publishers and editors — Brad Cummings, David Koechel, and John Peterson — played the roles of taskmasters, challengers, supporters, and invaluable contributors. Along the way, they became my friends. Thanks guys!

Dave Bohon has been an amazing editor who did so much more than I asked. He embraced this project as his own, and you, the reader, are the beneficiary of his commitment. Jon Godfredson provided impressive graphic designs and evocative visual enhancements which breathed a special strength into my words.

Cina Chapman relentlessly and skillfully scrutinized my manuscript for errors and ambiguities. Rita Hillman-Olson, Vicki Daley, and John Daly helped ensure that the book's central message did not detour from the concept that Big Pharma, Big Tech, and Big Government play a frightening role in determining what Americans see, hear, and talk about.

And finally, it is imperative that I acknowledge the ultimate source of energy necessary to get this project done. My patients, with their passion for truth and freedom and uncensored conversation, propelled this project.

You, the reader, have my eternal gratitude for consuming my words and standing up for liberty — yours and mine! You now have the opportunity to drive the dialogue that can forever change America's awareness of how Big Pharma, Big Tech, and Big Government combine to form a triad of tyranny. It is my prayer that you will help advance a national discussion on our healthcare system's shortcomings and demand nothing less than full disclosure of all things medical.

Without question, any errors or oversights herein are my doing and belong to me.

Scott Jensen, M.D.

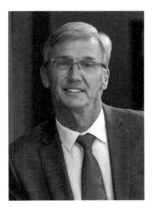

About the Author
Dr. Scott Jensen

I was born and raised in the quiet little town of Sleepy Eye, in the southern plains of Minnesota. It was a community in which safety was never an issue, and the entire village participated in raising its children. I was the middle child of five. Mom was my best friend, and Dad was my hero. Tragically, both my parents died young, and cancer became a lifelong enemy.

My career search took place on the heels of Mom's passing, and it wasn't a straight path. It included a year in dental school followed by a year in the seminary. A brief detour into the universe of law found me taking exams for law school, until I finally decided on medical school.

It was in the hallowed halls of hospitals that I fell in love with taking care of people, and this love affair has endured for forty years. Focusing on the physical, emotional, and spiritual aspects of my patients' well-being continues to provide me with immense joy and satisfaction. My patients bless me daily.

Hobbies are a necessary diversion from illness and suffering, and golfing, flying, writing, and skiing provide me with rejuvenation and thankfulness for an abundant life. Grandchildren are a relatively recent phenomenon, and they are a joy I could not have anticipated.

I live and practice medicine in the western suburbs of the Twin Cities, and I thank God for my lovely wife, Mary, and our three children. The blessings and growth Mary and I received from raising and loving our three kids go beyond the magic of mere words.

My years of doctoring have granted me complete confidence that departing this planet will lead to the ultimate journey of stepping over an earthly threshold into the realm of my Creator. I know I never stand alone, and daily I take great solace from the privilege of encountering my Maker through prayer.

In the midst of writing this book, my wife and I made a monumental decision that I would endeavor to be the next governor of Minnesota — not because such an adventure was on our mutual bucket list, but because the words of Esther 4:14 challenged both of us: "Have you considered you're in the position you're in, for such a time as this?"

My daily prayer is that I live better today than I did yesterday and that tomorrow I will do better still.

Life is a gift. Life is fragile. But above all, life is a rehearsal for the best which is yet to come. Count on it.

"Follow your conscience —

free from fear, coercion, and deceit.

Realize the power of shared voices.

And know this: alone, there is so

much we cannot do, but together,

there is so little we cannot do."

— SCOTT JENSEN